Alcohol Problems in Older Adults

Prevention and Management

Prevention and Management

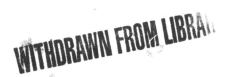

Kristen L. Barry, Ph.D., is a Senior Associate Research Scientist in the Department of Psychiatry and the Associate Director of the national Serious Mental Illness Treatment Research and Evaluation Center (SMITREC) for the Department of Veteran Affairs. She has a number of active and pending NIH and university-based grants. Dr. Barry's primary research foci include: alcohol problem detection and brief alcohol interventions in ambulatory care settings; relationships between substance abuse, mental health, and physical health functioning; treatment efficacy for adults with serious mental illness and co-occurring substance abuse disorders; women's alcohol use and mental health issues; and alcohol use by the elderly and related mental health issues.

David Oslin, MD, is an Assistant Professor of Psychiatry at the University of Pennsylvania Medical Center and the Philadelphia Veterans Affairs Medical Center. He holds joint appointments in the Section of Geriatric Psychiatry and the Center for Studies on Addiction. He completed residency training at the University of Maryland and fellowship training at the University of Pennsylvania. He is the recent recipient of a career development award from NIMH and is conducting research on the treatment of late life major depression that is complicated by other disorders such as alcohol dependence. He is also research on the treatment and consequences of alcohol dependence in older adults. He serves as an ad hoc reviewer for several journals and is a member of numerous professional and scientific societies.

Frederic C. Blow, Ph.D., is an Associate Professor and Senior Associate Research Scientist in the Department of Psychiatry at the University of Michigan and is Director of the National Serious Mental Illness Treatment Research and Evaluation Center (SMITREC) for the Department of Veteran Affairs, Ann Arbor, MI. His areas of research expertise including alcohol screening and diagnosis for older adults, serious mental illness and concurrent substance abuse, alcohol brief interventions in healthcare settings and mental health services research. Dr. Blow has been the principal investigator on numerous federal, state and foundation grants and has published extensively in the areas of substance abuse and alcoholism among the elderly, substance abuse screening/treatment and mental health. From 1996–98, Dr. Blow was Panel Chair for CSAT (Center for Substance Abuse Treatment) TIP (Treatment Improvement Protocol) on Substance Abuse Among Older Adults. Dr. Blow maintains an active role in both graduate and undergraduate teaching and the mentoring of pre- and post-doctoral students and junior faculty.

Alcohol Problems in Older Adults

Prevention and Management

Kristen Lawton Barry, PhD
David W. Oslin, MD
Frederic C. Blow, PhD

 SPRINGER PUBLISHING COMPANY

Copyright © 2001 by Springer Publishing Company, Inc.

Springer Publishing Company, Inc.
536 Broadway
New York, NY 10012-3955

Acquisitions Editor: Helvi Gold
Production Editor: Janice Stangel
Cover design by Susan Hauley

01 02 03 04 05 / 5 4 3 2 1

Library of Congress Cataloging-in-Publication-Data

Barry, Kristen Lawton
    Alcohol problems in older adults : prevention and management / Kristen Lawton Barry, David W. Oslin, and Frederic C. Blow.
        p. cm.
    Includes bibliographical references and index.
    ISBN 0-8261-1403-2
    1. Aged—Alcohol use.   2. Middle aged persons—Alcohol use.   3. Alcoholism—Treatment. I. Oslin, David W.   II. Blow, Frederic C.   III. Title.

    RC564.5.A34 B374 2001
    618.97'6861—dc21   00-052655

Printed in the United States of America by Capitol City Press

Contents

Preface

In the last two decades, information and knowledge has grown substantially regarding patterns of alcohol use and the consequences of at-risk use in older adulthood. We know now that the majority of older adults who experience physical, psychological, and social problems related to alcohol use do not meet criteria for alcohol abuse or dependence, and that the concepts and techniques presented here are useful when working with the majority of older adults who are experiencing problems related to their use of alcohol.

This manual is designed as a hands-on document and presents both the science and the art of the preventing and managing alcohol problems in older adults. It provids a guide to alcohol screening, assessments, and brief interventions, protocols for managing withdrawal, and a guide to referrals for more intensive care. The content is based on well-designed research, conceptual strides, and practical breakthroughs in this field. It presents the first systematic, practical approach to working in a variety of clinical settings with a growing population of vulnerable older adults who use alcohol at risk levels but often go unnoticed in everyday clinical practice. This book is designed for use in primary and specialty physical and mental health care settings by physicians, nurse practitioners, nurses, physician's assistants, social workers, psychologists, and case managers in older-adult facilities and programs. Although there is a growing body of information and research on the use and misuse of alcohol by older adults, we developed this book because there are very few practical references to assist clinicians with detection, prevention, and intervention strategies for older at-risk drinkers.

The book is divided into six chapters. The "Introduction and Background" is a concise overview of alcohol problems in later life. It includes definitions of low-risk drinking, at-risk drinking, problem drinking, and alcohol dependence; the risks and benefits of moderate drinking in this age group and prevalence estimates; and a review of the evidence regarding brief alcohol interventions. It also provides a synopsis of the most pertinent concepts and techniques needed to understand the extent of the problem, the potential comorbidities, and prevention and intervention methods.

Chapter 2, "Alcohol Screening," presents research and methods for alcohol screening in an older adult population. It covers questions about alcohol consumption (quantity and frequency of use); the Michigan Alcoholism Screening Test–Geriatric version (MAST–G) and the Short MAST-G (SMAST–G), an elder-specific alcohol screening instrument developed by Dr. Blow; the CAGE (a four-item screener for alcoholism); and the Alcohol Use Disorders Identification Test (AUDIT) developed by the World Health Organization and tested internationally. With older adults, it is often best to ask questions about alcohol use and its consequences in the context of other health behaviors (e.g. nutrition, exercise, smoking) and physical and mental health conditions (depression, cardiac, hypertension, diabetes). Alcohol screening questions can be asked in the following formats: interview, paper and pencil, computer, personal digital assistant, and Internet-based application. In most settings, the paper and pencil or interview. Paper and pencil are the most efficient and acceptable formats to older adults in busy clinical settings, leaving time to follow up with prevention or intervention messages when needed. Older adults who exceed the guidelines established by the National Institute of Alcohol Abuse and Alcoholism (NIAAA) (more than eight drinks a week; more than one drink a day) can benefit from brief, targeted alcohol advice or interventions to reduce or stop drinking.

In Chapter 3, "Brief Alcohol Interventions," the approach and workbooks are designed specifically for an older adult population and rely on concepts of motivational interviewing to enhance the commitment of older at-risk drinkers' to decrease or discontinue their drinking. The goal of intervention—either the reduction of use or abstinence—will depend on concurrent physical and mental health conditions, medications and on whether the older adult is ready to make a change. The brief intervention can elicit an immediate change or it can help the person assess usage and move closer to making a change. This section includes aspects of motivational interviewing, the administration of the initial brief alcohol intervention, possible follow-up sessions, and how to handle a number of issues that may occur when working with older patients. Although it is not possible to anticipate every situation, a thorough knowledge of the material contained in this book will provide clinicians with strategies to deal with unanticipated circumstances. Two useful workbooks are discussed in detail in this sectoin: *Health Promotion Workbook for Older Adults: Initial Session* and *Health Promotion Workbook for Older Adults: Follow-up Session.* Copies are included in Appendixes A and B. Samples of drinking diary cards for use during intervention are shown at Appendix C.

Methods and statements for handling a number of issues that are likely to occur during the course of the brief intervention are covered in Chapter 4, "Frequently Asked Questions." Among other issues, the section deals with resistance, steps in the management of older adults who are very heavy drinkers, responses to individuals who return to drinking at risk levels after reducing or stopping consumption, special confidentiality concerns, and depression and anxiety. The topics covered are based on collective clinical and research experience with older adults who are at-risk drinkers.

Chapter 5, "Special Circumstances," addresses alcohol withdrawal, concurrent benzodiazepine or opioid use, and strategies for working with very heavy drinkers. In the *Health Promotion Workbook for Older Adults: Initial Session,* discussed in Chapter 4 of this manual, older at-risk drinkers are asked if they have ever experienced withdrawal symptoms. If a history of withdrawal is reported, the likelihood of experiencing these symptoms again is increased when an individual is trying to cut down or stop drinking as part of the brief intervention protocol. Older adults who report a history of hospital-based detoxification or seizures should be monitored carefully during any attempt to cut down or discontinue alcohol use. an algorithm is included in this manual as an aid to determining the severity of withdrawal symptoms and to assist in the management of those patients with significant withdrawal symptoms.

The goal of this manual is to provide state-of-the-art, practical materials to detect, prevent, and intervene with older adults who are at-risk and problem drinkers. It is designed specifically to fit into busy clinical settings where time is of the essence and quality of care is critical. The decision was made to publish the appendices with a wider margin so that clinicians can photocopy easily the workbook that will be useful in their work with at-risk and problem drinking older adults.

Permission is granted by the authors to reproduce portions of this manual and the workbooks for noncommercial purposes. All reprints must bear the following copyright and credit line: Copyright © 2000 Kristen Lawton Barry, David W. Oslin, and Frederic C. Blow. Reprinted by permission.

We have moved into the 21st century with mandates to provide "best practice," guideline-driven care and at the same time to manage care in a cost-effective manner. Helping older adults who are at-risk drinkers to reduce or discontinue their use of alcohol is an excellent opportunity to improve the quality of their lives and to provide efficient state-of-the-art and best practice care. Because we are living longer than ever before, there is an increasing need to address prevention issues at every stage of life. It is possible to make a large difference with brief, targeted, systematic, nonjudgmental approaches to at-risk and problem alcohol use in an age group that we know can reap the benefits of small changes for years to come.

Kristen Lawton Barry
David W. Oslin
Frederic C. Blow

Acknowledgments

The authors wish to thank the University of Michigan Department of Psychiatry, the National Institute of Alcohol Abuse and Alcoholism (NIAAA), the Center for Substance Abuse Prevention (CSAP) and the Center for Substance Abuse Treatment (CSAT) for their support over the years for work on projects related to the content of this book. They also gratefully acknowledge the work and guidance of Michael F. Fleming, MD, MPH, Professor at the University of Wisconsin Department of Family Medicine, who conducted the first randomized clinical trials of brief alcohol interventions with younger and older adults in community-based primary care setting.

1

Introduction and Background

The brief alcohol intervention approach is designed specifically for an older adult population and relies on concepts of motivational interviewing to enhance patients' commitment to change their drinking. This manual reviews aspects of motivational interviewing, the administration of the initial brief alcohol intervention, possible follow-up sessions, and how to handle a number of issues that may occur when working with older patients who have alcohol use problems. It is not possible to anticipate every situation that can occur when working with older adults who are at-risk or problem drinkers. However, a thorough knowledge of the material contained in this manual will provide clinicians with strategies to deal with unanticipated situations.

This manual contains a review of a brief intervention aimed at reducing alcohol-related problems among older at-risk and problem drinkers as well as instructions for screening, administering the brief intervention, and conducting follow-up sessions. Information is also provided on frequently asked questions, special circumstances, and addressing the important issues of withdrawal, concurrent benzodiazepine or opioid use, and high levels of alcohol consumption. Appendixes are also included that contain instruments, workbooks, and information sheets. Although brief interventions have been studied for the most part in primary care settings, this manual can be used in a wide variety of clinical and nonclinical settings, including specialized addiction clinics and mental health clinics.

BACKGROUND

The promotion of health and prevention of primary disease among older adults is receiving growing attention as a larger proportion of the American population reaches late life. Record numbers of senior citizens are seeking costly health care for acute and chronic conditions. Because of their increased incidence of health problems, older adults are more likely, to seek care on a regular basis from their primary care providers than younger ones. Problem drinking can significantly affect a number of conditions in this age group, including depressive symptoms as well as general health functioning. Depression has been linked to relapse in drinking and increases in alcohol intake (Oslin, Katz, Edell, & TenHave, in press). Drinking has been shown to have an effect on general health, physical functioning, pain, vitality, mental health, role performance, and social functioning (Blow, 1998). It has been suggested recently that interventions targeted to lifestyle factors, including the use of alcohol, may be the most appropriate focus to maximize health outcomes and minimize health care expenditures among older adults.

One of the priorities in the Healthy People 2000 guidelines is to increase to at least 75% the proportion of primary care providers who screen patients for alcohol and drug use problems and provide counseling and referral as necessary. One of the challenges in meeting this goal within the context of a managed care environment—where providers are expected to deliver quality medical care for a wide variety of problems under greater time constraints—is the difficulty of addressing time-consuming activities that promote health. As more health care is delivered by managed health care organizations, the cost of treatment will decrease. At the same time the effectiveness of interventions for alcohol problems will increase because of innovative technologies that require less provider intervention time and are more targeted to each patient's particular set of symptoms and health patterns.

ALCOHOL PROBLEMS IN LATER LIFE

Despite significant advances over the last two decades in understanding of the aging process with its attendant health problems and in recognizing the consequences of alcohol problems and alcoholism, little attention has been paid to the intersection where gerontology, or geriatrics, and alcohol studies meet. In recent years, however, interest in alcohol problems among older people has increased. Although studies in this area are limited, prevalence estimates and typical characteristics of older problem drinkers have been reported. The *National Institute on Alcohol Abuse and Alcoholism (NIAAA) Drinking Guidelines for Older Adults* recommends the following for persons over the age of 65: no more than seven drinks per week (one drink per day); and never more than four drinks on any drinking day. (Alcohol use recommendations are generally lower than those for adults under the age of 65.)

Definitions

To understand the most effective types of alcohol interventions with older adults, it is necessary to define levels of alcohol use and discuss the consequences. For the purposes of this manual, *abstinence* refers to having ingested no alcohol in the previous year. A large percentage of older adults are abstinent, some because of a previous problem with alcohol. Some are abstinent because of a recent illness. Others have lifelong patterns of low-risk use (social drinking) or abstinence. It is important, therefore, that clinicians ascertain why the older adult is abstinent. Patients who have a history of alcohol problems may require preventive monitoring to determine if any new stresses could resurrect an old problematic drinking pattern.

It is important to note that some older adults who drink even small amounts of alcohol may experience alcohol-related problems. Older adults with certain chronic diseases such as diabetes or congestive heart failure, those taking medications that may interact with alcohol (e.g., benzodiazepines), those with psychiatric illnesses or more than mild cognitive deficits should be advised to abstain from drinking alcoholic beverages. The potential interaction of medication and alcohol, even in small amounts, is of great concern with this age group. For some clients, combining any alcohol at all with certain over-the-counter or prescription medications can increase negative health consequences.

Low-risk drinking is alcohol use that does not lead to problems. Persons in this category can set reasonable limits on alcohol consumption and do not drink when driving a motor vehicle or when using contraindicated medications. These persons can benefit from preventive messages but may not need interventions. For example, "Our goal is to prevent you from having additional health problems. Your walking program looks good and you have maintained your weight. Since you have no family history of alcohol or drug problems and are not taking medications that interact with alcohol, a glass of wine two to three times a week should not cause any additional problems for you at this time."

Drinking more than the recommended limits increases the chances that a person will develop problems and complications; this is called *at-risk drinking*. Although these patients do not have current health, social, or emotional problems because of alcohol, they may experience family and social problems, and if this drinking pattern continues, health problems could be exacerbated. These older adults can benefit from a brief alcohol intervention.

Older adults engaging in *problem drinking* are consuming alcohol at a high enough level to have resulted in adverse medical, psychological, or social consequences. Potential consequences can include accidents and injuries, medication interaction problems, and family problems, among others. In addition to quantity and frequency of alcohol use, it is important to determine whether the patient has experienced any common alcohol-related consequences. The presence of consequences, even if drinking levels are below guidelines, should drive the need for intervening.

Alcohol or drug dependence refers to a medical disorder characterized by loss of control, preoccupation with alcohol or drugs, continued use of alcohol or drugs despite adverse consequences, and physiological symptoms such as tolerance and withdrawal. Research indicates that people with alcohol dependence can benefit from brief interventions, which can be focused either on alcohol consumption or on issues related to alcohol problems such as a specific family issue or entry into specialized alcoholism treatment.

Risks and Benefits of Moderate Drinking in Older Adults

Before discussing the negative consequences of drinking in late life, it is important to review the beneficial effects of moderate drinking, which are being used to promote moderate alcohol consumption among otherwise healthy older adults, especially with regard to cardiovascular disease and mortality (Kadden et al., 1995; Klatsky, Armstrong, & Friedman, 1990; Rimm et al., 1991; Stampfer, Colditz, Willett, Speizer, & Hennekens, 1988). Findings from the cardiovascular literature has led to a host of articles in the popular press espousing the benefits of alcohol use and has also led some people to recommend alcohol consumption to persons who formerly did not drink. More recent epidemiological studies have also suggested a protective effect of moderate alcohol use in reducing the risk of demental illness and cancer (Broe et al., 1998; Orgogozo et al., 1997). Several authors have also demonstrated that among older non-institutionalized persons, moderate alcohol use of less than one drink per day is associated with fewer falls, greater mobility, and improved physical functioning when compared to a comparison group of nondrinkers (LaCroix, Guralnik, Berkman, Wallace, & Satterfield, 1993; Nelson, Sattin, Langlois, DeVito, & Stevens, 1992; Nelson, Nevitt, Scott, Stone, & Cummings, 1994; O'Loughlin, Robitaille, Boivin, & Suissa, 1993).

It is also widely accepted that alcohol is consumed socially and may help to reduce stress in social situations (Dufour, Archer, & Gordis, 1992). Moreover, alcohol in moderate amounts may improve self-esteem or provide relaxation. A more recent study of moderate and heavy drinking among older adults found that the low levels of alcohol consumption on a near daily basis were not associated with poor psychosocial functioning, thus indirectly supporting the effects of responsible drinking that are not harmful (Graham & Schmidt, 1999). In contrast, higher levels of alcohol consumption per day regardless of the frequency (so-called binge drinking) did lead to poorer psychosocial functioning.

Given the beneficial effects of drinking and in the absence of alcohol dependence or heavy drinking, it is not surprising that clinicians and the public at large may be confused about recommendations to change or reduce consumption—or even possibly to initiate it—for therapeutic effects. Clinicians may know that a patient is in fact having two to three drinks a day; but they may be unaware of the risks associated with that level of drinking in an older adult, and thus would make no provision for treatment. While there are benefits moderate drinking, the practice of recommending drinking to people who currently do not drink is not advocated. Many older adults do not drink because of past problems or family problems with drinking, because of the expense or the unpleasant effects of intoxication, or simply because they do not like the taste. There is no evidence to support the therapeutic effect of alcohol for heart disease or any other condition in persons who did not drink previously. For a summary of the risks and benefits, see Appendix D.

Excess Physical Disability in Older Adults

The physical effects of alcohol on older adults are much more of a general health concern than in a younger population. Higher blood alcohol concentrations, coupled with an increased breakdown of the blood-brain barrier and aging body systems are not as well equipped can result in greater medical morbidity at lower levels of consumption in older compared to younger adults. Several studies support this vulnerability and have demonstrated the harmful health effects of drinking more than one standard drink per day or seven per week. At-risk drinking of more than seven drinks per week has been shown to increase the risk of stroke caused by bleeding, although it decreases the risk of stroke caused by blocked blood vessels (Hansagi, Romelsjo, Gerhardsson, Andreasson, & Leifman, 1995). At-risk drinking has also been demonstrated to impair driving skills and leads to other injuries such as falls and fractures (Council on Scientific Affairs, 1996; Kivela, Nissinen, & Ketola, 1989). The risk of breast cancer has been shown to increase by approximately 50% in women who consumed three to nine drinks per week compared to women who drank fewer than three drinks per week (Willett et al., 1987). Of particular importance to older adults is the potential harmful interaction between alcohol and prescription and over-the-counter medications, especially psychoactive medications such as the benzodiazepines, barbiturates, and antidepressants. Alcohol is also known to interfere with the metabolism of many medications such as digoxin and warfarin (Adams, 1995; Fraser, 1997; Hylek, Heiman, Skates, Sheehan, & Singer, 1998). With regard to physical functioning, a history of alcohol use doubles the impairment to basic activities of daily living among older women (Ensrud et al., 1994). In fact, alcohol use was more strongly correlated to impairment than smoking, age, the use of anxiolytics, stroke, or grip strength.

Older adults who consume more than an average of four drinks per day or whose drinking has led to a diagnosis of alcohol dependence are at the greatest risk for excessive physical disability and physical illness related to the drinking. Alcoholic liver disease, chronic obstructive pulmonary disease (COPD), peptic ulcer disease, and psoriasis are the most common problems observed in older alcohol-dependent patients. A current or lifelong history of alcohol use can also lead to significant mental health problems in older adults. Findings from the Liverpool Longitudinal Study found a fivefold increase in psychiatric illness among older men who had a history of five or more years of heavy drinking (Saunders et al., 1991). Comorbid mental disorders that have a particular association with alcohol use include anxiety disorders, affective illness, cognitive impairment, schizophrenia, and antisocial personality disorder.

The effects of moderate or at-risk alcohol consumption on mental health disorders are of special interest. In a recent study of more than 2,000 patients, Oslin and colleagues demonstrated an added benefit of reducing low levels of alcohol use while treating a depressive disorder (Oslin et al., in press). This study defined moderate alcohol use as one to seven drinks per week and further demonstrated that the higher the alcohol consumption, the greater the negative effect on the treatment of depression. At least three studies have found that people who have primary major depression with comorbid alcoholism experience more severe symptoms, are less likely to show improvement of depressive symptoms, and have a greater chance for suicide compared to subjects with secondary depression (Hasegawa, Mukasa, Nakazawa, Kodama, & Nakamura, 1990; Schuckit et al., 1997; Tsuang, Cowley, Ries, Dunner, & Roy-Byrne, 1995). Sleep disorders and sleep disturbances represent another group of comorbid disorders associated with excessive alcohol use. It is well established that alcohol causes changes in sleep patterns such as decreased sleep latency, decreased stage IV sleep, and precipitation or aggravation of sleep apnea (Wagman, Allen, & Upright, 1977). There are also age-associated changes in sleep patterns including increased REM episodes, decreases in REM length, stage III, and IV sleep, and increased awakenings, which can all be worsened by alcohol use.

Extent of the Problem

Prevalence estimates of problem drinking among older adults using community surveys have ranged from 1% to 15% (Blow, 1998). These rates vary widely depending on the definition of risk drinking (alcohol abuse or dependence) and the methodology used in obtaining samples. Among clinical populations, however, estimates of alcohol abuse or dependence are substantially higher because problem drinkers of all ages are more likely to present themselves in health care settings.

Rates of concurrent alcoholism have been reported at 15% to 58% among older patients seeking treatment in hospitals, primary care clinics, and nursing homes for medical or psychiatric problems (Blow, 1998). Most older patients are not recognized as problem drinkers by health care personnel. Because the role of physicians and other health care professionals may be crucial in identifying those in need of treatment, improved, efficient identification of older at-risk and problem drinkers during health-seeking encounters has great potential value.

Studies of Brief Alcohol Intervention

Alcohol interventions for older adults range from prevention and education for persons who are abstinent or low-risk drinkers to minimal advice or brief structured interventions for at-risk or problem drinkers to formalized alcoholism treatment for drinkers who meet the criteria for abuse or dependence. The last is generally used with persons who cannot or do not discontinue drinking after a brief alcohol intervention.

Low intensity, brief interventions have been suggested as a cost-effective and practical technique for initially approaching problem drinkers in primary care settings. The last two decades have seen an increased interest in conducting controlled clinical trials to evaluate the effectiveness of early identification and secondary prevention using brief intervention strategies for treating problem drinkers. This is especially important for those with relatively mild to moderate alcohol problems who are potentially at risk for developing more severe problems.

Studies on brief alcohol intervention have been conducted in a wide range of health care settings, from hospitals to primary health care locations to mental health clinics. Individuals recruited from such settings are likely to have had some contact with a health care professional over the course of study participation, and therefore alcohol-related professional assistance presumably was available. Nonetheless, many or most of these patients would not have been be identified by their health care provider as having had an alcohol problem and therefore would not ordinarily receive any alcohol-specific intervention. Even if identified and referred, heavy drinkers are the least inclined to seek formal alcoholism treatment.

A number of large randomized controlled trials of brief alcohol interventions with younger adults have found significant differences between treatment and control groups. The following are key examples of major studies to date.

The World Health Organization Project was undertaken at international collaborating centers in 10 countries, including the United States (Babor & Grant, 1992). Male ($n = 1,362$) and female ($n = 299$) subjects recruited from hospitals, primary care clinics, work sites, and educational settings were randomly assigned to three conditions: control, simple advice, or brief counseling. Few older individuals were included, and those over the age of 70 were generally excluded from the study. At a minimum six-months' follow-up, there were significant effects of both interventions on various alcohol consumption measures for male subjects, with an approximately 25% reduction in daily consumption in the treatment group compared with the control group. In addition, after accounting for spontaneous improvement in the control group for men (42% reduced drinking by one standard drink or more), an additional 21% of both intervention groups reduced their drinking. Indications were that women in the intervention groups, especially those under the brief counseling condition, improved more when comparing percentages of change. Finally, the intensity of the intervention—simple advice versus brief counseling—did not have a differential effect on drinking behavior: Five minutes of brief advice was as effective at reducing consumption as a more extensive counseling session.

The Trial for Early Alcohol Treatment (Project TrEAT) was the first randomized clinical trial in the United States to test the effectiveness of generic brief physician advice on problem drinkers between the ages of 18 and 64 in community-based primary care settings (Fleming, Barry, Manwell, Johnson, & London, 1997). The study was conducted in 17 primary care practices in 10 counties in southern Wisconsin, and the 64 community-based physicians participating in this trial were family physicians and internists. Patients were asked to complete a five-minute screening. Of a total of 17,695 patients screened, 1,705 participated in a face-to-face assessment. A total of 482 males and 292 females reported drinking above the limits set for the trial and were randomized into a control ($n = 382$) or intervention group ($n = 392$). Subjects in Project TrEAT were followed up in 12 months. The follow-up rate at 12 months was 92%, and at that time there was a significant reduction in seven-day alcohol use, in episodes of binge drinking, and in frequency of excessive drinking in the treatment group compared with the control group. The relative difference in alcohol use between the groups at 12 months was 17% in the male sample and 34% in the female sample. A twofold significant difference in inpatient hospital days was noted in the intervention group compared with the control group.

Extending Brief Alcohol Interventions to Older Adults

Little attention has been given to brief alcohol intervention research for older adults, who present unique challenges in applying these strategies for reducing alcohol consumption. The level of drinking that is considered risk behavior is lower for older adults than for younger individuals. Intervention strategies need to be nonconfrontational and supportive due to the greater shame and guilt experienced by many older problem drinkers. As a result, older adult problem drinkers find it particularly difficult to identify their own risky drinking. In addition, chronic medical conditions may make it harder for clinicians to recognize the role of alcohol in decreased functioning and quality of life in their patient. These issues present barriers to conducting effective brief alcohol interventions for this vulnerable population.

The objective of two recently elder-specific studies of brief alcohol intervention was to determine the efficacy of brief advice in reducing alcohol use and health care utilization in older adult, at-risk, and problem drinkers. Project GOAL: Guiding Older Adult Lifestyles was a randomized, controlled clinical trial conducted in Wisconsin with 24 community-based primary care practices (43 practitioners) located in 10 counties (Fleming, Manwell, Barry, Adams, & EA., 1999). Of the 6,073 patients screened for problem drinking, 105 males and 53 females met inclusion criteria ($n = 158$) and were randomized into a control ($n = 71$) or intervention group ($n = 87$). One hundred forty-six subjects participated in the 12–month follow-up procedures. The intervention consisted of two 10–15 minute, physician-delivered counseling visits, which included advice, education, and contracting using a scripted workbook. No significant differences were found between groups at baseline on alcohol use, age, socioeconomic status, smoking status, rates of depression or anxiety, frequency of conduct disorders, lifetime drug use, or health care utilization. Project GOAL found that there was a significant reduction in seven-day alcohol use ($t = 3.77$; $p < .001$), in episodes of binge drinking ($t = 2.68$, $p < .005$), and frequency of excessive drinking ($t = 2.65$, $p < .005$) at the 12–month follow-up, providing some of the first direct evidence that physician intervention with older adult problem drinkers decreases alcohol use and health resource utilization in the U.S. health care system.

The second and larger elder-specific study is the Health Profile Project currently underway in primary care settings in southeast Michigan (Blow & Barry, in press). The intervention contains brief advice discussion by a psychologist or social worker, as used in the WHO studies, and motivational interviewing techniques including feedback. The study included 44 primary care clinics (with 13 predominately primarily minority clinics) and screened more than 14,000 older adults. Of these, 6% of patients have screened positive for alcohol problems based on alcohol consumption. A total of 460 subjects were randomized with more than 26% African Americans. The 12-month follow-up rate is 96%. Preliminary results in the Health Profile Project compared baseline with 3–month follow-up binge-drinking outcomes. There was a significant reduction in binge drinking for the intervention groups when compared with the control group ($F = 50.59, p < .0001$), suggesting that the elder-specific generic brief intervention is particularly useful in reducing the dangerous effects of binge drinking in a vulnerable older population.

Brief alcohol intervention studies to date support recommendations that early identification, screening, and brief interventions should be a matter of routine practice in primary care settings to detect patients with hazardous or harmful patterns of alcohol use (M. Fleming, 1999). This is especially important for older adult patients, given their unique vulnerabilities. Early identification and secondary prevention that is directed in straightforward, non-technical terms to older adults who are likely to be motivated to change could have broad positive public health implications. It appears that brief alcohol interventions consisting of one or a few sessions have the potential of reaching the largest number and broadest spectrum of older individuals from diverse settings (M. Fleming, 1999).

2

Alcohol Screening

To conduct prevention and early intervention with older adults, clinicians need to screen for at-risk and problem alcohol use and for interaction problems between alcohol and medication. Screening can be part of routine mental and physical health care and should be undertaken annually, or before the older adult begins taking any new medications, or in response to problems that may be alcohol-or medication-related. This manual recommends a combination of quantity and frequency questions, a binge-drinking question, and the Short MAST–G to provide a comprehensive alcohol screening test for older adults.

Because of the relationship between alcohol consumption and health problems, questions about consumption (quantity and frequency of use) provide a method to categorize patients into levels of risk from alcohol use. The traditional assumption that all patients who drink have a tendency to underreport their alcohol use is not supported by research. If asked in a sensitive and nonjudgmental manner, people who are not alcohol dependent generally give accurate answers to questions about alcohol use. Clinicians can get more accurate histories by asking questions about the recent past, embedding questions about alcohol use in the context of other health behaviors (i.e., exercise, weight, smoking), and by paying attention to nonverbal cues that suggest the patient is minimizing use (i.e., blushing, turning away, fidgeting, looking at the floor, changes in breathing pattern). In patients with mild or moderate cognitive impairment, spouses or other family members are also valuable informants.

Screening questions can be asked in a person-to-person interview, by paper-and-pencil or computerized questionnaire, or by telephone interview. All four methods are equally reliable and valid. Any positive responses should lead to further questions about consequences. To successfully incorporate alcohol (and other drug) screening into clinical practice, it should be simple and be consistent with other screening procedures already in place.

Before asking any screening questions the following conditionsmust be met: (a) the interviewer should be friendly and nonthreatening; (b) the purpose of the questions should be clearly related to the patient's health status; (c) the patient should be alcohol-free at the time of the screening; (d) the patient should be informed that the information they provide will be kept confidential; and (e) the questions must be easy to understand. In some settings (such as waiting rooms), screening instruments are given as self-report questionnaires, with instructions for the patient to discuss the meaning of the results with their health care provider. It should be remembered that not all patients can see well enough to complete questionnaires or read at a level necessary to complete questionnaires. Alcohol screening for older adults also can be conducted successfully by telephone interview.

If the alcohol questions are embedded in a longer health interview, a transitional statement is needed to move into the alcohol-related questions. The best way to introduce questions about alcohol is to give the patient a general idea of the content of the questions, their purpose, and the need for accurate answers. The following is an example of such an introduction: "Now I am going to ask you some questions about your use of alcoholic beverages during the past year. Because alcohol use can affect many areas of health and may interfere with certain medications, it is important to know how much you usually drink and whether you have experienced any problems with your drinking. Please try to be as accurate as possible."

This statement should be followed by a description of the types of alcoholic beverages typically consumed: "By alcoholic beverages we mean your use of wine, beer, vodka, sherry, and so on." If necessary, include a description of beverages that may not be considered alcoholic such as cider and low-alcohol beer. Determinations of consumption are based on "standard drinks." A standard drink is a 12 oz. bottle of beer, a 4 or 5 oz. glass of wine, or a 1½ oz. shot of liquor such as vodka, gin, whiskey. When using standardized screening questionnaires in an interview, it is important to read the questions as written and in the order indicated for better comparability between your results and those obtained by other interviewers.

Appendix D contains questions for determining alcohol quantity and frequency. The Screening Questions are general questions, and the Assessment Questions are more specific. These provide greater specificity about drinking and are not prone to the underreporting errors that are made when patients have to report their average consumption over time. This method also mirrors the drinking diary cards used in the brief intervention and can be used to track a patient's alcohol use over time.

In addition to determining the quantity and frequency of drinking, a number of screening instruments have been developed to probe for problems related to alcohol use. The following section provides background on three screening instruments that are used with older adults: the Michigan Alcoholism Screening Test–Geriatric Version (MAST–G); its shortened version, the SMAST–G; and the widely known CAGE questionnaire. Appendix E describes other typical screening and assessment questions and ones for benzodiazepine or opioid use.

The Michigan Alcoholism Screening Test–Geriatric Version (MAST–G) was developed by Dr. Blow and colleagues at the University of Michigan as an instrument for use with older adults in a variety of settings. Psychometric properties of this instrument are superior to other screening tests for identifying older persons with alcohol abuse or dependence. The MAST–G was the first major elderly-specific alcoholism screening measure to be developed with items unique to older problem drinkers.

The MAST–G has a sensitivity of 94.9%, specificity of 77.8%, positive predictive value of 89.4%, and negative predictive value of 88.6%. Similar values were found after excluding those subjects who do not currently drink. Therefore, psychometric properties were stable when considering only those who had an opportunity to meet criteria for a current diagnosis.

The Short Michigan Alcoholism Screening Test–Geriatric Version (SMAST–G) (see Appendix F) is the short form of the MAST–G and was developed for use in busy clinical settings where the length and administration time of the longer scale major barriers to using it. To address these issues, a short version of the MAST–G was developed. The SMAST–G fared as well as the Alcohol Use Disorders Identification Test (AUDIT) and is more acceptable to older individuals. The SMAST–G is also an acceptable alternative to the MAST–G for elder-specific brief alcohol screening and is superior to other screening instruments developed in younger populations. A score of two or more (e.g., two "yes" responses) indicates probable alcohol problems. The SMAST–G asks about patients' experiences within the last year. If responses are ambiguous or evasive, continue asking for clarification and ask the patient to choose the response closest to their experience. Recording the drinking pattern can be difficult if the patient does not drink on a regular basis. For example, if the patient was drinking heavily in the one month before an accident but has not had any alcohol since, it will not be easy to characterize the "typical" drinking pattern. The amount of drinking and related symptoms for the heaviest drinking period of the entire past year will provide the most useful information. However, clinicians need to make a note of the special circumstances and time period assessed for that particular patient.

The CAGE is the most widely used alcohol problem screening test in clinical practice. It contains four items regarding alcohol use: the desire to to Cut down on drinking, being Annoyed that people have criticized one's drinking; feeling Guilty because of criticism about one's drinking; and having an "Eye-opener," a drink upon waking in the morning to get rid of a hangover. Two positive responses are considered a positive screen and indicate that further assessment is warranted. The sensitivity and specificity of the CAGE varies from 60% to 90% and from 40% to 90% respectively (Buchsbaum, Buchanan, Welsh, Centor, & Schnoll, 1992; Ewing, 1984). Among older adults, using a score of one positive does improve the sensitivity without lowering specificity. However, older adults who do not screen positive on the CAGE may still have problems with alcohol use. For instance, they may not have been annoyed by others about their drinking because family members may not know or they may not have close contact with friends. In addition, very few older adults need an eye-opener upon waking or they may consume alcohol at a level they used when younger and not believe they need to cut down. On the other hand, older women are more likely to say they feel guilty evcen when using very little alcohol.

The Alcohol Use Disorders Identification Test (AUDIT) is well validated in adults under 65 in primary care settings (Babor & Grant, 1992; Saunders, Aasland, Babor, Delafuente, & Grant, 1993) and has had initial validation in a study of older adults (Jones, lndsey, Yount, Soltys, & Farani-enayat, 1993; Morton, Jones, & Manganaro, 1996). The AUDIT is comprised of two sections: a ten-item scale with alcohol-related information for the *previous year only,* and a Clinical Screening Procedure, which includes a trauma history and a clinical examination. The questionnaire is introduced by a section explaining to the respondent that questions are included about alcohol use in the *previous year only.* The questionnaire is often used as a screener without the clinical examination. The recommended cut-off score for the AUDIT has been 8, but Blow et al (Blow, 1998) found a Cronbach's alpha reliability of 0.95, sensitivity of 0.83, and a specificity of 0.91 in a sample of older adults with a cut-off score of 7.

Biological markers of alcohol use have proved to be a less accepted measure in clinical practice but can be useful. There are several laboratory values such as a blood alcohol level or an acetate level, which is a metabolite of alcohol, that indicate recent use or abuse (Salaspuro, 1994). Long-term markers of disease include the following: gamma-glutamyl transferase (GGT) which has a low sensitivity and a moderate specificity for diagnosing an alcohol use disorder; mean corpuscular volume, which has a low sensitivity but a high specificity; high density lipoprotein (HDL), which shows a linear increase with alcohol use; and carbohydrate-deficient transferrin (CDT), which has a moderate sensitivity and moderate specificity (D. W. Oslin, et al., 1998). For medications and drugs of abuse, urine drug screens continue to be useful as both a screening tool and as a confirmation of self-report. The majority of drugs of abuse will remain detectable in a urine drug screen for 4 or more days and some for several weeks.

3

Brief Alcohol Interventions

REVIEW OF MOTIVATIONAL INTERVIEWING

This manual and intervention were developed specifically for older adults seen in primary care settings. Thus, the intervention addresses issues such as the effects of alcohol on health and body systems, the reasons older adults may have problematic drinking patterns, how the modification of alcohol use can specifically benefit them, and the methods to change their drinking habits.

This brief alcohol intervention approach is based on the concepts of effective brief interventions including the *FRAMES* model developed by Miller and Rollnick (1991). The FRAMES model identifies key elements that have been shown in previous research to be effective in assisting persons with at-risk or problem drinking to change their drinking behavior.

Motivational interviewing is an approach to discussing an older patient's problems, concerns, and ambivalence about their drinking and to help the individual recognize the risks associated with their level of alcohol use. It is especially useful when patients are reluctant or ambivalent about changing their drinking and enables the older adult to make the decision to cut down or stop drinking alcohol. It is a supportive, respectful approach that is persuasive without being coercive or cajoling and is particularly relevant in working with older patients.

Elements of Effective Brief Alcohol Interventions

The FRAMES model is a guide for thinking about how to approach older drinkers using the workbook and methods included in this manual. The following table describes the elements of the FRAMES model specific for older adults.

Feedback	• providing useful feedback based on screening to the older at-risk or problem drinker (one who drinks more than over recommended limits)
Responsibility	• the focus of changing drinking is the personal responsibility of the older adult, not the clinician (negotiated change)

Advice	• providing the older adult with specific recommenda-tions for changing drinking (to drink below weekly recommended limits)
Menu	• offering options for the older adult so that change in drinking is more likely to occur (reduction in drinking versus abstinence)
Empathy	• showing an understanding of the older adult's goals and the role of alcohol in his or her life to help moti-vate change (for example, "I can see how you would feel that way")
Self-Efficacy	• validating the older adult's confidence in changing his or her drinking ("I think you can do this, too.")

Differences Between Confrontational Approaches and Motivational Interviewing

Motivational interviewing differs in a number of ways from many tradi-tional approaches to modifying problematic behaviors. For example, a com-mon method of attempting to assist people in modifying their alcohol use is to employ a confrontational approach aimed at removing obstacles to chang-ing drinking behavior. Although some people may benefit from such an approach, research confrontation is particularly problematic with older adults who may be experiencing shame and guilt about their drinking. Fur-thermore, a confrontational approach is not a necessary aspect of alcohol intervention or treatment and may actually increase defensiveness, denial, or treatment dropout, which may be harmful to a substantial proportion of older adults with alcohol problems.

Motivational interviewing differs from confrontation in substantive ways. In particular, motivational interviewing avoids the use of labels such as alcoholic; emphasizes personal choice and responsibility for change; focuses on eliciting patients' own concerns; understands that the role of the clini-cian can effect the level of resistance in the patient; uses reflection to meet resistance; and engages in the negotiation not the prescription of drinking goals and strategies. Motivational interviewing is an approach that can avoid certain aspects of interpersonal interactions that can sidetrack a discussion or reinforce resistance to change.

General Instructions for Administering the Brief Alcohol Intervention

Brief alcohol interventions follow general guidelines that include "setting the scene," use of the structured workbook to facilitate the intervention, summary or "end game" of the initial session, and the use of follow-up sessions to enhance persons' motivation to change and meet their drinking goals.

- It is important to establish a supportive setting conducive to the intervention.
- Interventions should be conducted in private rooms separate from family and other staff.
- Begin by introducing yourself if needed.
- Thank patients for completing the screening and brief assessment.
- Explain that you want to go over the results of the screening as it relates to their health and well-being.
- Sit next to older adults with the workbook between you so that you can work on this together. A table or a clipboard can be used.
- Explain that you will be using a workbook as part of the discussion. The workbook is a guide to talk about a variety of health issues.
- Explain that the workbook is theirs to keep and refer to as often as they would like.
- The person conducting the intervention will write in the book during this meeting. Information provided in the screening questionnaire, as well as that provided during the session, will be written in the workbook by the clinician.
- Personalize the workbook by writing the patient's name on the first page. Put the date of the intervention in the top right corner of the first content page.

The purpose of the workbook is to provide a guide for the clinician on key points to address with patients and key issues to elicit from patients. You need to cover each part of the workbook, although you may not address every item. All the elements throughout the workbook are meant to stimulate patients to think of their specific concerns and issues.

Proceed through the Step-by-Step Brief Alcohol Intervention in this chapter. The entire intervention should take no longer than 15 minutes. At the end of the initial intervention session, provide a brief summary of the discussion points and the decision made regarding drinking goals. Make an appointment with the patient for a follow-up visit in 6 weeks. Encourage patients to use the workbook, the drinking diary cards, and to call with any questions or concerns.

Follow-up sessions can enhance the persons' ability to meet their goals. However, many people in studies of brief alcohol interventions make changes in their drinking without returning for specific follow-up visits. Follow-up visits should occur at 6 weeks and 12 weeks after the initial intervention session and are an opportunity to provide a check-up on progress toward meeting drinking goals. Barriers, risky situations, and strategies for change are reviewed in these follow-up sessions.

Brief intervention protocols often use a workbook containing the components listed below, steps 1 through 9. The workbook contains sections for the patient and clinician to complete on drinking cues, reasons for drinking, reasons to cut down or quit, a drinking agreement in the form of a prescription, and drinking diary cards for self-monitoring. The approach to patients is non-confrontational and generally follows motivational interviewing principles as described by Miller and Rollnick, which were reviewed earlier in this chapter (Miller & Rollnick, 1991).

INITIAL BRIEF INTERVENTION SESSION

This section contains instructions for reviewing the workbook with patients. The instructions in this manual will focus on how to review the Initial Session Workbook with older adults, keeping in mind the basic tenets of motivational interviewing. Due to the uniqueness of each individual older adult patient and their reactions to the materials covered, it will be necessary for clinicians to deal with responses in a flexible manner. The review of motivational interviewing at the beginning of this booklet should serve as a guideline for how clinicians react and respond to patients. However, there are also some general reminders or suggestions throughout the instructions for ways of dealing with some of the more easily anticipated patient responses. It is important to be familiar with all aspects of this manual, so please review it in depth.

Following the identification of at-risk or problem drinkers through screening techniques, a semistructured brief intervention can be conducted. The content of the intervention needs to be elder-specific and includes the following:

Step-by-Step Brief Alcohol Intervention

Step 1: Identifying Future Goals for Health, Activities, Hobbies, Relationships, and Financial Stability

Identifying future goals is important for many older adults, because it establishes a context for thinking about the role of drinking in their lives. This part of the intervention establishes rapport and begins to focus patients' attention on a future orientation. This helps to set the context for the brief intervention and generally provides increased motivation for the individual to change.

Key Points:

• Discuss how the older person would like his or her life to improve and be different in the future. This helps develop a discrepancy between what patients desire in their life and how their current drinking behavior may negatively impact those goals.

• It is important to elicit from the older person the goals that are most important, not to cover all areas. For example, some people may not have goals for their financial situation but will choose goals related to their physical health or living situation.

• When people respond with stating they have no goals, give some examples such as maintaining their current health and independence, improving a chronic health problem, or maintaining contact with family or friends.

Dialogue Example:

"What are some of your goals for the next 3 months to a year regarding your physical and emotional health, your activities and hobbies, your relationships and social life, and your financial situation and other parts of your life?"

Step 2: Summary of Health Habits

Customized feedback on screening questions relating to drinking patterns and other health habits may also include smoking, nutrition, tobacco use, and so on. The summary is in the form of a health profile on screening questions relating to drinking patterns and other health habits. This information could be derived from screening and preassessment or from the patient during this session.

Key Points:

• Summarize information on other health behaviors *first*.
• After reviewing the alcohol section of the health habits portion of the workbook, ask the patient if there are any health behaviors with which they would like help. Generally, patients will not indicate alcohol use as a targeted health behavior. Patients often ask for help with another health behavior (i.e., exercise, nutrition). This gives the clinician the opportunity to move the patient toward a discussion of alcohol by briefly offering assistance with those behaviors and then moving to a discussion of alcohol.

Dialogue Example:

"I'm pleased that you are interested in exercise and nutrition. That's great! These are important areas. I can set up a time for you to talk with the nutritionist [or other]. Right now, I'd like to discuss your use of alcohol with you."

"You indicated that, on average, you drink alcohol almost every day and that you drink one to two drinks at a time."

Step 3: Introduce the Concept of Standard Drinks

This discussion focuses on the equivalence of alcohol content among various beverage types, which provides the context for a discussion of sensible drinking limits. In addition to determining quantity and frequency of use, it is important to ask about the size of the beer container, glass of wine, and the amount of liquor in a typical drink. For example, a patient who drinks wine in a water glass may be consuming more than one "standard drink" at a time, but may think of it as one drink.

Key Points:

• The following examples are roughly equivalent in alcohol content: 12 oz. of beer or ale; 1.5 oz. of distilled spirits; 5 oz. of wine; 4 oz. of sherry or liqueur.

• When pouring wine, sherry, or distilled spirits, measuring is important to ensure that the patient is consuming standard drinks.

• Alcohol is alcohol, though some patients may think that they do not use alcohol because they "only drink beer or wine." Some differentiate between hard and soft alcoholic beverages becasuse of their effects.

• Review standard drinks briefly. Avoid disputes about picky details regarding the alcohol content of specific beverages.

Dialogue Example:

"Did you know that a 12 oz. beer, 5 oz. of wine, and 1½ oz. of liqueur all contain the same amounts of alcohol?" [show the equivalent figure.]

Step 4: Discuss the Types of Older Drinkers in the Population and Where the Patient's Drinking Patterns Fit Into the Population Norms for His or Her Age Group

(Remember: One standard drink = 12 oz. of beer or ale; 1.5 oz. of distilled spirits; 5 oz. of wine; 4 oz. of sherry; 4 oz. of liqueur.)

The purpose of this section is to introduce the idea that patients' alcohol use can be related to their physical and emotional health, and that their level of drinking can put them at risk for more health-related problems.

Key Points:

• Review the graph of how much other people drink. Point out that their level of drinking is not typical of others their age and that most older people drink less that they do.

• Review this material in a matter-of-fact manner.

• This section may evoke a number of strong reactions from patients (argumentiveness, minimization, acceptance, concern, tearfulness, embarrassment, hostility).

• It is important to avoid creating additional resistance. It is very important to roll with the patients' resistance or reluctance in order to examine further their drinking behavior in an empathetic manner.

Dialogue Examples:

"National guidelines recommend that men your age drink no more than seven drinks per week; no more than one per day. Your pattern of alcohol use fits into the at-risk drinking category."

"From what you've said, I can see that you do not consider yourself as fitting into the at-risk and problem drinking category. Let's just say you are more than a light drinker and look at some of the things that can happen at your level of alcohol use."

Step 5: Consequences of At-Risk and Problem Drinking

This section addresses reasons for drinking and weighing the benefits and drawbacks of drinking. This is particularly important because the clinician needs to understand both the positive and negative role of alcohol in the context of the older patient's life, including coping with loss and loneliness. This section is also designed to facilitate patients' understanding the potential social, emotional, and physical consequences of drinking. This is an important aspect of motivational interviewing. It provides a climate in which patients can obtain greater clarity of how alcohol is or could be negatively affecting their lives.

Key Points:

• Some older patients may experience problems in physical, psychological, or social functioning even though they are drinking below cut-off levels.
• Note that some of the things on the list were problems they indicated they were having. Other items are common problems people could have if they continued their current drinking practices.
• Maintaining independence, physical health, and mental capacity can be key motivators in this age group.
• Some patients may minimize how alcohol contributes to their problems. Again, roll with resistance, don't argue with it.

Dialogue Examples:

"We've spent some time talking before about your sleep problems, your blood pressure problems, the fall you took in the bathroom, and your loneliness since your wife died."

"Even though your drinking is close to the limit for people your age and you drank at this level for years, I am concerned about some of the health problems you've had and about your loneliness."

"I am concerned that the amount you are drinking could be making some of these problems worse. Our goal is for you to remain as independent as possible and have a good quality of life."

"Although alcohol use has been linked to such problems, you have to evaluate the situation yourself. Whether to be concerned about the potential consequences of drinking heavily is your decision."

It should be noted that some patients may begin to recognize that their drinking is problematic. Try to elicit motivational statements with evocative questions: *"In what way does this concern you?" "What do you think will happen if you don't make a change?"*

Step 6: Reasons to Quit or Cut Down on Drinking

This is a discussion of how changing drinking levels could benefit the individual. Some older patients may experience problems in physical, psychological, or social functioning even though they are drinking below cut-off levels. This section reviews the potential social, emotional, and physical benefits of changing their drinking.

Key Points:

• Maintaining independence, physical health, and mental capacity can be key motivators in this age group.
• Be careful not to promise miracles or cures. Alcohol use is often a component of health problems not the sole etiology.
• Before moving to the next section, you should make an effort to elicit self-motivational statements.
• Strategies that are useful in this age group include developing social opportunities that do not involve alcohol, getting reacquainted with hobbies and interests from earlier in life, and pursuing volunteer activities if possible.

Dialogue Example:

"From what you've said, you are really concerned about being able to continue living in your own house. There are a number of things that you can do to help to maintain your independence. Cutting back on your drinking is one important thing you can do."

Step 7: Drinking Agreement

Agreed-upon drinking limits that are signed by the patient and the clinician are particularly effective in changing drinking patterns. The purpose of this section is for the patient to choose a goal (moderation or abstinence) and to complete the agreement.

Key Points:

• Give guidance on abstinence versus cutting down. Complete the contract. Be sure to allow patients to decide which plan they prefer.
• Patients who have a serious health problem or who take medications that interact with alcohol should be advised to abstain.

• Others may be appropriate candidates for cutting down on drinking to less than recommended limits.

• Provide guidance by recommending a low level of alcohol use or abstinence. Remember that you may have to negotiate up, so start low.

• The drinking agreement is in the form of a "prescription."

• The prescription-type form contains space for writing what you have negotiated with patients:

> to stop or cut down on drinking
> when to begin
> how frequently to drink
> for what period of time

• If patients are reluctant to sign contracts, try to determine the reason for their reluctance and alleviate their concerns if possible.

• Be sensitive to patients' reactions including concern, embarrassment, defensiveness, minimization of drinking problems, or hostility. Here again, it is very important to roll with the patients' resistance or reluctance in order to examine further their drinking behavior in a matter-of-fact and empathic manner. Avoid disputes over these guidelines and whether they agree with them or not, ask that they be patient and continue with the strategies to see how alcohol could affect their life.

Dialogue Examples:

"I would suggest that you drink no more than three days a week, no more than one standard drink on any drinking day. What do you think about that level of alcohol use?"

"I see that you like to have a bottle of beer each night with dinner. You can do that as long as you drink no more than one 12 oz. bottle of beer a day."

"I am concerned about your hypertension and how difficult you say this is to control. Given this, I would recommend that you abstain from alcohol now. What do you think of this recommendation?"

"It is up to you to decide if you should do anything about your drinking. I would still like to review the rest of the workbook with you. You may find some of it helpful, and if you decide to make some changes this might be useful. Just take what you can use and leave the rest."

Step 8: Coping With Risky Situations

Social isolation, boredom, and negative family interactions can present special problems in this age group. This section is aimed to help patients identify situations and moods that are related to drinking too much alcohol and to identify some individualized cognitive and behavioral coping alternatives.

Key Points:

• Work with patients to develop strategies to deal with such issues as social isolation and negative family interactions.

• It is important to encourage patients to come up with their own alternatives and to provide minimal guidance as necessary.

• Remind patients that by providing individualized feedback, the intervention is concerned with their unique situations.

• Review at least one roadblock and solution, and review the rest as you have time. Role-playing specific stressful situations can be helpful and will vary depending on patients' particular situations.

• Remember that motivation to change occurs as the perceived benefits of change outweigh the reasons for drinking (the barriers to change).

Dialogue Example:

"You've said that one of the reasons you drink more than the recommended limits is that you are lonely since you retired and your wife died you have nothing to occupy your time. You also have said that you and your wife used to play cards at the senior center. Have you thought about going back to the senior center to start doing some of the things you like to do there?"

"Sometimes quitting or cutting back on drinking involves making some very difficult decisions, like not getting together with certain friends or not going to certain places like the bar or club. You should think about the kinds of things that would be just as rewarding for you to participate in."

"You say that you drink because you enjoy meeting your friends at the bar. Have you considered other places where you could meet these friends or how you might meet some new friends?"

Step 9: Summary of the Session

The summary should include a review of the session, including a review of the agreed-upon drinking goals, a discussion of the drinking diary cards (calendar) to be completed for the next 6 weeks, and the recommendation to refer back to the workbook materials given to patients during intervention sessions.

Key Points:

• The tone of the summary should be empathetic, encouraging, and positive.

• Review the drinking diary cards. Tell patients that you have additional cards when these are filled.

• Make a final effort to elicit self-motivational statements.

• Give an appointment card for the 6-week follow-up session.

• Thank patients for their time and cooperation.

Dialogue Example:

"We've covered a lot of material today and you've done really well in identifying how alcohol has been affecting your health and how continued drinking above limits can make your health conditions worse. You have a good plan for cutting down on your drinking. I know that you can reach your goal of drinking no more than one drink a day."

"Sometimes people have days when they drink more than they thought they would. Just record the number of drinks you had on the drinking diary card. Don't be discouraged. Start over the next day following the limits we set together."

ELICITING MOTIVATIONAL STATEMENTS AND ENHANCING COMMITMENT TO CHANGE

The purpose of this section is to provide additional examples of statements patients may make that indicate a willingness to work on reducing or stopping their drinking and of motivational statements that you can use to facilitate the change. The concepts underlying these statements are adapted from Miller and Rollnick (Miller & Rollnick, 1991).

A critical aspect of the intervention is eliciting motivational statements from patients. Table 3.1 is an example of these statements and suggested responses. It is the clinician's task to facilitate the patients' expression of their reasons for changing their drinking as well as their resolve to change. Motivational statements tend to fall into four categories: problem recognition, expression of concern, openness to change, and optimism. It is important to reinforce statements that indicate a willingness to consider change. The use of evocative questions can help elicit motivational statements and enhance the commitment to change. Furthermore each motivational statement may help patients realize that the benefits of changing outweigh the costs.

FOLLOW-UP SESSIONS

This section contains instructions on how to review the follow-up workbook with patients. In general, the same tenets of motivational interviewing are to be used for follow-up interviews including being as flexible and supportive as possible. When conducting a follow-up session, two principles should be kept in mind. First, you have already had an initial session with the patient, which will allow more emphasis or focus on alcohol consumption and its consequences during follow-up. Second, the timing and frequency of follow-up sessions are dictated by clinical needs. In general, it is recommended that a follow-up session be conducted 6 weeks and 12 weeks after the initial session.

The purpose of follow-up sessions can be multifaceted. Foremost, you are showing concern about the patient; thus follow-up sessions are a method for

Table 3.1
Examples of Motivational Statements and Evocative Statements

Type of Statement	Patient's Statement	Evocative Questions
Problem recognition	I guess there is more of a problem than I thought.	What other problems have you had?
	I never realized how much I was drinking or what the recommended drinking limits were for people my age.	What else have you noticed or wondered about?
	I always thought I could drink the same amount I drank when I was younger.	How does knowing the limits change how you feel about your drinking?
Expression of concern	I'm a little worried about this. I really feel bad about letting this happen.	What other concerns have you had? What else worries you about your drinking?
Openness to change	I think it's time for me to think about quitting.	What are some other reasons you may need to make a change?
	I guess I need to do something about this.	Do you have any ideas about what you can do?
	This isn't how I want to be. What can I do?	Well, it is different for everybody. What do you think you can do that would help?
Optimism	I think I can change my drinking.	A positive outlook is very important. Why else do you think you can succeed?
	I'm going to overcome this. Now that I've decided, I'm sure I can change.	

emphasizing your concern about patients, their health, and the consequences of patients' alcohol consumption. The sessions also serve the function of assisting patients in monitoring their behaviors. This needs to be done in a compassionate and helpful manner, not in a parental or confrontational manner. The follow-up sessions are also an opportunity to support patients' efforts in changing their behavior. Finally, these sessions are an opportunity to give direction or to advise how to maintain or improve upon patients' goals.

Step-by-Step Follow-up Alcohol Intervention

Step 1: Purpose of Visit

It is important to identify to the patients the reason they have returned for this visit. This part of the intervention builds rapport and establishes the tone of the visit.

Key Points:

 • Let patients know you will be reviewing their alcohol consumption since the last time you saw them.
 • This is a time to let patients know that you will be reviewing their experiences with adhering to their drinking goals.
 • Let them know that you will be reviewing their drinking goals together and deciding whether these goals need revising or modifying.

Dialogue Example:

"Thank you for coming back today. The reason I asked you to come in was for us to see how you are doing with the goals you set around your alcohol use. I would like to review with you how much you are drinking currently and look at your drinking goals to see if you want to change them in any way or if you need any further help in maintaining these goals."

Step 2: Review of Alcohol Use

This section is used to review patients' alcohol consumption since their last visit. You may have two sources of information for this section: the patient's drinking diaries and self-report. The purpose of reviewing their current drinking is to assess and assist patients better. This review is not meant to be punitive or confrontational, and you should be nonjudgmental about whether patients met their goals. Reviewing drinking habits can be enlightening for patients in terms of realizing how much they are drinking or how well they are doing in cutting down.

Key Points:

 • If patients have brought in drinking diaries, review them and summarize the amount they are drinking. Translate the drinking records to standard drinks when necessary.
 • Look for trends in patterns since the last time you met.
 • Ask about drinking during the previous week and record this in the workbook.

Dialogue Example:

"Did you find using the drinking diary cards useful? Let's look at the ones you have brought with you."

"Now let's talk about last week. Did you have any drinks this past week?"

Step 3: Review of Changes in Alcohol Use

This discussion focuses on patients' efforts to change. You will first make observations about whether there were changes in drinking based upon diary information, then patients will indicate if they believe they are meeting their goals. Finally, this is the opportunity to listen to patients about what it was like to try cutting down. You want to hear successes as well as struggles. Listening at this point will be crucial to developing ideas on how to improve or maintain the goals.

Key Points:

• Establish if there has been any change in consumption since the last meeting based upon diary records.
• Get a feel from patients about their goals and if they feel they are meeting them.
• Listen to patients tell how they achieved their goals or struggled with achieving their goals.

Dialogue Example:

"Based on the last week of drinking, it looks like you have decreased your drinking since the last time we met. That's impressive. How do you think you are doing in terms of the goal you set for yourself?"

"Based on the last week of drinking, it looks as if you have increased your drinking since the last time we met. How does your current drinking match the goal you have for yourself?"

"What was it like to think about or try changing your drinking patterns? Did you find it hard or easy?"

Step 4: Consequences of At-Risk and Problem Drinking

This section addresses the reasons for drinking and weighs the benefits and drawbacks of drinking. This section is designed to facilitate the patients' understanding of the potential social, emotional, and physical consequences of drinking. Linking any changes in drinking to change in other aspects of life is important for maintaining behavioral modification. As discussed in Step 5 of "Step-by-Step Brief Alcohol Intervention" above (p. XX), this provides a context in which patients can see with greater clarity of how alcohol is or could be negatively affecting their lives. During your dialogue with patients you can begin to understand what changes are occurring in their livers relative to their drinking.

Key Points:

• Some older patients may experience problems in physical, psychological, or social functioning even though they are drinking well below cutoff levels.

• Maintaining independence, physical health, and mental capacity can be key motivators in this age group.

• Some patients may minimize how alcohol contributes to their problems. Listen, but don't argue. Look for opportunities to point out the possible relationship between drinking and disability.

Dialogue Examples:

"Even though your drinking is close to the limit for people your age and you drank at this level for years, I am still concerned about some of the health problems you've had and about your loneliness."

"We spoke last time about how drinking affects your sleep. Have you noticed any change in your sleep since then?"

"I am concerned that the amount you are drinking could be making some of these problems worse. Our goal is for you to remain as independent as possible and have the best quality of life that you can."

Step 5: Reasons to Quit or Cut Down on Drinking

This section starts to focus on an individual's motivation for change. Maintaining behavioral changes can be very difficult, as anyone who has tried to diet is well aware. Although there may have been some very important events or situations that have made the patient decide to cut down on alcohol, the reasons may get lost over time, and this can lead to a lapse back into old habits. Moreover, some patients may take weeks or months to come to the decision to modify their behavior, and some may not come up with any reasons during the initial session but may at the follow-up session. During this time with patients, you want to listen for the things that are important to them and link those to how alcohol may be affecting them. This section reviews the potential social, emotional, and physical benefits of changing their drinking.

Key Points:

• When appropriate, link a reduction in alcohol use to their maintaining independence and function.

• Highlight positive changes and improvements that have already occurred.

• Strategies that are useful in this age group include developing social opportunities that do not involve alcohol, getting reacquainted with hobbies and interests from earlier in life, and pursuing volunteer activities if possible.

Dialogue Example:

"You indicate that you are still concerned mostly about your health. As we discussed, cutting back on your drinking is one positive thing you can do that may improve your health. You have been doing a really good job of cutting back on your drinking, and I would encourage you to continue with your goal."

"The last time we met I suggested that drinking may be affecting your overall health. Have you given this any further thought? Is there something that would motivate you to reduce you alcohol use?"

Step 6: Drinking Agreement

Agreements to limits drinking that are signed by patients and by the clinician are particularly effective in changing and maintaining drinking patterns. The purpose of this section is for patients to choose a goal—moderation or abstinence—and to complete the agreement. The goal can be the same as that established in a prior session or a new goal. Reaffirming goals that have been achieved is also important.

Key Points:

* Provide guidance on abstinence versus cutting down. Complete the contract. Be sure to allow patients to decide which plan they prefer.
* Patients who have a serious health problem or who take medications that interact with alcohol should be advised to abstain.
* Others may be appropriate candidates for cutting down on drinking to less than recommended limits.
* Provide guidance by recommending a low level of alcohol use or abstinence. Remember that you may have to negotiate up, so start low.
* The drinking agreement is in the form of a "prescription."
* The prescription-type form contains space for writing what you have negotiated with patients:

    stop or cut down on drinking
    when to begin
    how frequently to drink
    for what period of time

* If patients are reluctant to sign contracts, try to determine the reasons for their reluctance and alleviate their concerns if possible.
* Be sensitive to patients' reactions including concern, embarrassment, defensiveness, minimization of drinking problems, or hostility. It is very

important to roll with patients' resistance or reluctance in order to examine further their drinking behaviors in a matter-of-fact and empathic manner. Avoid disputes over these guidelines and suggest that they continue to monitor for benefits and consequences of drinking. Never try to force your opinions about drinking limits when they are directly in conflict with those of the patients.

Dialogue Examples:

"You last set a goal of cutting back to eight drinks per week, I would suggest that you now consider no more than 3 days per week, with no more than one standard drink on any drinking day. What do you think about this new goal?"

"Now that you have cut down to two drinks every day, what do you think about a new goal?"

"When you were here last time, we had set a goal of one drink per day. Although you did not meet that goal, I think it is important to renew your goal. As you found out, trying to moderate drinking is sometimes harder than eliminating alcohol altogether. Perhaps you might try abstinence as a goal for the next several months."

Step 7: Coping With Risky Situations

Social isolation, boredom, and negative family interactions can present special problems in this age group. This section is aimed at helping patients identify situations and moods that are related to drinking too much alcohol and to identify some individualized cognitive and behavioral coping alternatives.

Key Points:

   • Work with patients to develop strategies for dealing with such issues as social isolation and negative family interactions.
   • Discuss the strategies that were used since the last time you met.
   • Probe for mood or anxiety problems and consider additional treatment if these are present.
   • Review at least one roadblock and solution, and review the rest as you have time. Role-playing specific stressful situations can be helpful. The role-play exercises will vary depending on patients' particular situations.
   • Remember that motivation to change occurs as the perceived benefits of change outweigh their reasons for drinking (the barriers to change). Thus the amount of time and energy needed to address each risky situation cannot be greater than the time and energy it takes to drink.

Dialogue Example:

"You stated that since retiring your getting together with friends is an important part of the reason you drink. Can you think of some ways you can get the compan-

ionship you want but not in a setting that involves drinking? Are there activities that you enjoy that don't involve drinking?"

"You said that you tried going to a senior center and church but you didn't feel like you fit in. Are there places that you would enjoy going to?"

Step 8: Summary of the Session

The summary should have a review of the session, including a review of the agreed-upon drinking goals, a discussion of the drinking diary cards (calendar) to be completed for the next several weeks, and the recommendation to refer back to the workbook materials given to patients during intervention sessions. If you are going to be getting together for another visit, you should discuss when this will occur.

Key Points:

   • The tone of the summary should be empathetic, encouraging, and positive.
   • Review the drinking diary cards. Tell patients that you have additional cards to use when these are filled.
   • Make a final effort to elicit self-motivational statements.
   • Give an appointment card for the next session.
   • Thank patients for their time.

Dialogue Example:

"We've covered a lot of material today and you've done really well in identifying how alcohol has been affecting your health and how continued drinking above limits can worsen your health conditions. You have a good plan for cutting down on your drinking. I know that you can reach your goal of drinking no more than one drink a day."

"Sometimes people have days when they drink more than they thought they would. Just record the number of drinks you had on the drinking diary card. Don't be discouraged. Start over the next day, following the limits we set together."

4

Frequently Asked Questions

This section contains instructions for handling a number of issues that are likely to occur during the course of the intervention. It is important to rely on some general methods for dealing with these issues since they may occur at any time during the intervention.

1. How do I deal with a resistant patient?

Resistance can happen at any point during the intervention and can manifest itself in many different ways. *It is often a signal that the clinician is not using strategies appropriate for the patient's current stage of change.* In general, the best way of responding to resistance is with nonresistance. Acknowledging the patient's disagreement, emotion, or perception allows for further exploration and discussion.

2. How do I respond when patients contest the accuracy, expertise, or integrity of the clinician?

When patients directly challenge the accuracy of what the clinician has said, it is most likely to occur during the feedback portions of the intervention. It is possible that patients may benefit from additional information about the material in the booklet. For example, it may be helpful to reiterate that the material in the booklet is based on studies with adults their age and to provide a little more detail to address their questions or challenges, which can also include a discussion of the limitations of the material presented in the booklet. In addition, acknowledging that the information may or may not apply to them can be helpful in reducing disputes about minor details.

Example of response:
1. "You feel that this doesn't really apply to you. Maybe it doesn't, and that's fine. Let's take a closer look to check it out either way. You are the expert on you, so you'll know better than I do."
2. "Take what you find helpful, and leave the rest. You will be better able to decide if this applies to you than I will."

A patient's expressing hostility toward the clinician can happen at any time during the intervention, especially during the feedback portions. It is important to acknowledge patients' anger and to express openness to their concerns and feelings. Reflective listening can help diffuse anger and hostility. You may also wish to inform patients that you don't want them to be angry and that you are very interested in what they agree *and* disagree with.

Example of response: "Sounds like you're pretty angry with me. You're the expert about your situation. Tell me what you disagree with." [utilize reflective listening]

It is possible that patients may become angry and say something like, "You're saying I'm an alcoholic," or "I'm not an alcoholic, and this is none of your business." In these situations, it is still important to acknowledge their anger, to be open to their concerns, and to use reflective listening. However, it is also important to de-emphasize labels since they tend to increase resistance. Let patients know that you are not concerned with labeling them in any way and reflect their concerns.

Example of response: "I don't really care for labels like that, and it seems that you don't either. I don't blame you, I wouldn't want to be labeled either. I'm just concerned about whether or not drinking is harming you in any way and what you might want to do about it if it is. The bottom line is, its up to you to decide if this is something you want to do something about.

3. How do I respond when the patient denies there is a problem or refuses to cooperate?

When the patient expresses an unwillingness to recognize his or her problems, cooperate, accept responsibility, or take advice it will most likely occur during the feedback sections of the intervention (see Survey Responses and Types of Drinkers, the Pros and Cons, and the Drinking Agreement and Plan sections).

The patient suggests that the clinician is exaggerating the risks and that really isn't so bad. It is important to let patients know that it is up to them to decide what information is relevant to them.

Example of response: "You realize you've occasionally had some problems associated with your drinking, but you say that you're not doing so badly. It is up to you to decide how serious your problems are and whether you should do anything about them."

When patients claim they are not in any danger due to their drinking, it is most likely to occur during the discussion of the types of drinkers and pros and cons sections.

Example of response: "You are correct. I cannot say for sure if some of
                        your current·problems [or medical conditions] will
                        get worse because of drinking. Other adults of your
                        age and gender who drink about the same as you
                        either have some problems related to drinking or
                        are likely to have problems in the future. No one
                        knows for sure what will happen. You have to
                        weigh the pros and cons for yourself and decide
                        how much risk you are willing to live with."

If the patient firmly expresses a lack of desire or an unwillingness to
change or an intention not to change, it will most likely happen during the
drinking agreement and plan phases.

Example of response: "That is completely up to you. You should do what
                        you think is best. If you feel differently in the fu-
                        ture or run into some problems, you may find this
                        booklet helpful. I would still like to get together
                        with you in several weeks to see how your health
                        is."

It is important to avoid the arguing trap in this situation. However, we
still want to review all of the materials with patients so you may wish to
state the following:

Example of response: "What I would like to do is to go through the rest
                        of the booklet, to give you an idea of what is in it.
                        You've told me what you plan to do, and that is
                        okay with me. What I would like you to do is to
                        consider whether any of this may be helpful to you
                        and to tell me what you don't think is helpful about
                        the booklet."

4. Does the patient need to become completely abstinent to be successful?
    In general, the answer to this question is no. Success is measured not by
the patient achieving abstinence but rather by reaching a drinking level
that is appropriate for the individual. Abstinence should be the goal in patients with abusive or dependent drinking or when patients suffer from
other health problems such as hypertension or pulmonary disease that are
exacerbated by even moderate drinking. However, in the absence of alcohol-related problems or chronic medical problems, the goal may be simply
to get the at-risk drinker to become a moderate drinker.
    5. How do I deal with a really heavy drinker?
    Heavy drinking is associated with greater risks to patients and therefore
requires greater attention. There is a further discussion of heavy drinking
and potential adjunctive treatments in Chapter 5.

6. What do I do when someone returns to drinking after successfully reducing or quitting?

The response is to be empathetic. The initial goal is to reengage patients, to schedule follow-up visits, and to assess their needs. Use the follow-up workbook to structure this time.

Example of response: "I am glad you have come in to see me. You say that you have increased your drinking. Let's talk about the success you had in cutting down before and whether you want to set a new drinking goal for yourself."

7. When is drinking okay for an older adult?

This question is often asked in the context of information about the beneficial effects of alcohol on cardiovascular disease. Studies have strongly suggested but not proved that moderate drinking can reduce the risk of cardiovascular disease. While some of these studies have included older adults, most were conducted on relatively healthy people in their 50s and 60s. There are no studies to show that increasing or initiating drinking is helpful or wise when cardiovascular disease is present. In general, older adults who are otherwise healthy should enjoy alcohol in a responsible manner. However, if there are chronic medical problems or if the person is taking medications that are affected by alcohol, then abstinence may in fact be the better choice.

8. How can family members help?

Involvement of family member can be helpful in terms of supporting patients' goals. However, as with any mental health condition one needs to be aware of confidentiality. See question #9 in this section for further discussion of confidentiality. As for including family in the treatment sessions, we would recommend that the majority of time be spent with the patient alone. If patients want to review the goals with their family members, it can be done at the end of sessions. Allowing a family member to enter the session at the end also allows for engagement in the treatment plan rather than limiting the session to a personal health review.

If family members are to be involved, there are a number of ways they can be supportive or be included in the treatment. They can assist patients in traveling to the appointments, in removing alcohol from the residence, in filling in the diary cards, and by being empathetic to patients' goals. The clinician should exercise caution in having the family member monitor alcohol use as this can be construed by the patient as overly parental. However, with more cognitively impaired patients or patients who want this level of involvement family monitoring may in fact be reasonable.

9. How do I get other clinicians to refer patients and to support the need for treatment?

When working in settings such as outpatient mental health clinics, primary care office, or other medical sub-specialty clinics, it is important that all the providers support the need for screening and intervention. Otherwise, patients will not be referred to you for treatment and your credibility will be undermined in terms of establishing drinking goals. However, this may be difficult because identifying patients without demonstrated illness and conducting a treatment is sometimes counter to modern medicine as the evidence of the beneficial effects of moderate drinking mounts. Unfortunately, many clinicians consider moderate drinking anything less than three or four standard drinks per day or anything short of alcohol dependence. Fortunately, there is an increased awareness of the need for preventive medicine and for targeting preventive interventions. A good example would be conducting cholesterol screening and treating those with elevated levels as a way to prevent cardiovascular disease.

The real importance of this issue is the need to be prepared in advance and to spend time educating and negotiating how brief interventions will be conducted in a particular clinic. This includes ways in which to communicate findings, intervention goals, and outcomes with the other providers either through progress notes or verbal communication. When conducting interventions in clinic settings, it is useful to provide in-service education periodically for the other providers and office staff. You can use examples of patients from that clinic who were successful in reducing their drinking as a reminder of how this can be on appropriate treatment.

10. How do I assess for alcohol withdrawal?

Alcohol withdrawal can be a life-threatening emergency, patients should always be watched for potential withdrawal symptoms. For a full discussion of alcohol withdrawal, please see Chapter 5.

11. Are there any special confidentiality issues about patients who drink?

Clinicians should exercise extreme caution regarding the release of medical records, verbal or written. This arises when family members call to ask about patients or step in at the end of sessions. Prior to any discussion with family members, the clinician and patient should agree on what information can be divulged and to whom. The person performing the intervention should also be clear about whom information is to be shared with including the patient's primary care physician if this intervention is performed in a primary care setting. Similar issues and guidelines arise with employers, friends, and other health professionals.

12. What should I say if patients ask if they are expected to go to AA?

The answer is no. Self-help groups can be extraordinarily important for some people, but these groups are not for everyone. Older adults may be especially put off by self-help groups. Many groups include few older peers and involve participants who are polysubstance abusers. Moreover, for at-risk or moderate drinkers the idea of a self-help group may further alienate them from wanting to participate in the intervention because they do not feel they should be labeled an alcoholic.

13. The patient seems to be depressed or have anxiety. How do I manage this?

The connection between alcohol and depression and anxiety is complex. Alcohol can cause depression and anxiety or can be a reaction to the presence of depression or anxiety. Key steps include assessing the level of distress and deciding what steps should be taken to address it. Measuring symptoms of anxiety of depression can be done with any of a number of standardized instruments including the Hamilton Rating Scale for Depression; the Hamilton Rating Scale for Anxiety; the Center for Epidemiologic Studies—Depression Scale; the Beck Anxiety Scale; or General Health Questionnaire (Goldberg, 1978; Hamilton, 1960; Radloff, 1977; Schwab, Bialow, Clemmons, & al, 1967). In treating patients for alcohol problems, be careful not to ignore symptoms that don't meet diagnostic criteria, as these depressive or anxious symptoms can have significant impact on treatment outcomes for drinking. Because the intervention manuals do not include formal assessments for anxiety or depression, the clinician will need to use clinical judgment in deciding whether to assess for these problems. It may be appropriate to depart from the brief intervention protocol to assess the level of depression or anxiety in patients who are known to be depressed or who identify these symptoms early during the intervention. Of particular concern here is the combination of suicidal ideation and either depression or drinking. Both depression and drinking are strongly associated with completed suicide especially in older adults. The presence of moderate or severe depression or heavy drinking should always be followed by questions regarding suicide risk.

The next step is to decide what level of intervention is necessary for addressing the patient's distress. For patients with only a few or mild symptoms, the treatment may be to focus on reducing the alcohol use and watchful waiting with regard to the depressive or anxiety symptoms. For more distressing symptoms or in patients who meet syndromal diagnoses for a depressive or anxiety disorder, treatment may include pharmacotherapy or more formal psychotherapy.

A key in treating patients who present with more complex symptoms is to recognize your own limitations for providing care and to seek assistance through consultation or referral.

14. When should I refer a patient to a psychiatrist or specialty addictions program?

Some patients with more severe problems or patients who do not respond well to the recommendations found in this manual may need services found in more traditional specialty addiction programs. These services might include more formalized detoxification programs, group therapy, and case management or formalized psychotherapy. In addition, you may need consultative help from a psychiatrist or other mental health specialist for patients with complex symptoms such as comorbid depression or anxiety. You should use a consulting provider to help with complex diagnostic problems or when using medications with which you are not familiar.

There are two important considerations when referring patients to other providers. First, referrals are conducted either to assist in the management of the patient or as a consultation. Thus, referrals are usually made when the patient is not meeting the goals and you are unable to provide enough or the right services to meet these goals. There is generally no need to refer patients automatically just because they meet certain criteria such as concurrent depression. Second, it is important to consider whom you are referring to and your continued role in the patient's care. In considering referral sources for older patients, take into account the patient and the referral site. Patients may have special circumstances such as transportation or mobility problems or financial problems that limit where they can go for care. As for the referral sources, try finding local and regional resources that have a track record for caring for older adults.

Finally, do not think of referral as the end point. Stay connected with the patient; continue to conduct follow-up sessions using the workbook. This is supportive, empathetic and gives the patient their best chance of success.

5

Special Circumstances

ALCOHOL WITHDRAWAL

Overview

Alcohol withdrawal symptoms commonly occur in patients who stop drinking or markedly cut down their drinking after regular heavy use. Alcohol withdrawal can range from mild, nearly unnoticeable symptoms to severe and life-threatening ones. The classic symptoms associated with alcohol withdrawal include autonomic hyperactivity (increased pulse rate, increased blood pressure, increased temperature), restlessness, disturbed sleep, anxiety, nausea, and tremor. More severe withdrawal can be manifested by auditory, visual, or tactile hallucinations, delirium, seizures, and coma. Although withdrawal symptoms are likely to last longer in older adults and withdrawal potentially may complicate other illnesses, there is no evidence to suggest that these patients are more prone to alcohol withdrawal or that they need longer treatment for withdrawal symptoms.

Although alcohol withdrawal delirium is a life-threatening situation, serious problems are preventable and, when present, are usually manageable. Most patients are able to reduce or stop drinking with only minimal withdrawal symptoms. This module is designed to identify patients who are experiencing significant alcohol withdrawal symptoms and to outline the management of these patients.

Course of Alcohol Withdrawal Symptoms

There is no way of knowing whether alcohol withdrawal symptoms will occur and to what degree. However, the course of withdrawal symptoms is rather predictable. Within 6 hours of stopping or markedly reducing alcohol intake, withdrawal symptoms tend to be minimal if present at all. From 6 to 24 hours, symptoms begin to emerge such as tremor, nervousness, malaise, palpitations; elevations in heart rate; blood pressure, and temperature; sweating, nausea, anorexia, and sleep disturbances. These symptoms usually peak in severity within 24 to 36 hours and subside within 48 hours. In more severe cases, patients may experience withdrawal seizures and hallucinations or become delirious. These symptoms most often occur between 36 and 72 hours after cessation of drinking. Thus, in terms of evaluating a patient for withdrawal symptoms and the need for treatment, the clinician must know the time of the last drink or the time that the person dramatically reduced his or her drinking. Someone who has not used alcohol for more than 3 to 4 days should not be at risk for suddenly developing withdrawal symptoms. One final note here is that in addition to acute withdrawal effects, alcohol does cause more enduring effects that are also disturbing to patients such as disrupted sleep patterns and changes in attention and concentration. These effects may take days or months to reverse and should not be treated in the same manner as acute withdrawal.

When to be Concerned about Alcohol Withdrawal

There are few absolutes in terms of predicting who will suffer alcohol withdrawal symptoms and who will not. As a general rule, however, alcohol withdrawal symptoms are more likely to occur in patients who dramatically reduce or stop their drinking after regularly using large quantities of alcohol. Withdrawal symptoms are thought to occur because of substantial changes in blood alcohol levels that effect the nervous system. In practical terms, this means that patients who become abstinent after daily use of more than three or four drinks per day are more at risk for withdrawal. This does not mean that patients who drink less than this will not experience withdrawal symptoms, and you should be mindful of this possibility.

Often the patient is the best source of information about the potential for withdrawal symptoms. Many, if not most, patients have had occasion to cut down or stop drinking for one reason or another. During these times, patients may have had withdrawal symptoms and can describe them to you. If patients report alcohol withdrawal symptoms in the past, they are likely to experience these symptoms again when cutting down or quitting. Patients who reportedly need to be hospitalized for detoxification or report having had seizures should be carefully monitored when trying to reduce their alcohol use.

In the initial workbook, patients are asked if they ever experienced withdrawal symptoms when not drinking. You can use this question to probe further the severity of past withdrawal symptoms and the need for treatment.

Withdrawal Assessment and Management Algorithm

Figure 5.1 shows an algorithm that we have developed as an aid to determining the severity of withdrawal symptoms among older outpatients and to assist in the management of those with significant withdrawal symptoms. This algorithm has been formulated by consensus and has not been empirically tested, therefore, clinicians should rely on sound clinical judgment in cases with which you are uncomfortable and for concerns not addressed by the algorithm.

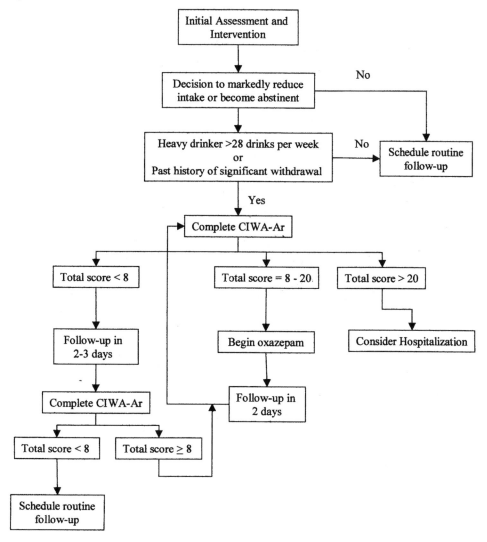

FIGURE 5.1 Alcohol Withdrawal Management Algorithm

When to Use the Algorithm

When screening and assessing patients in an outpatient setting, you should consider three factors in determining the potential for a patient's to suffering withdrawal symptoms. The first factor is quantity of alcohol consumption. Patients who are infrequent or moderate drinkers are less apt to suffer withdrawal symptoms or, if they do, to experience only mild symptoms. The second factor is withdrawal symptoms that generally occur only when patients dramatically reduce or eliminate their alcohol consumption. Gradually tapering alcohol use does not usually cause significant withdrawal effects. Based on these facts, it may be presumed then that no one should attempt going "cold turkey," but rather that patients should taper their alcohol use over time. However, trying to *cut down* rather than *stop* is not likely to be successful for those individuals who are alcohol dependent or who have high craving states. Thus, the dilemma is that those who are at the highest risk for withdrawal symptoms are the very ones who would probably be successful by eliminating alcohol use rapidly under medical supervision (e.g., detoxification). The third factor is history of previous withdrawal symptoms. Patients who have had previous withdrawal symptoms are more inclined to manifest symptoms again, possibly because they are somehow vulnerable to them and because the presence of withdrawal symptoms is an indication of greater alcohol use.

We recommend that persons with the following clinical characteristics be followed up according to the algorithm: (a) the patient is currently drinking more than 28 drinks per week; and (b) the patient's goal is to eliminate or markedly reduce his or her drinking; or (a) the patient reports a past history of significant withdrawal symptoms; and (b) the patient's goal is to eliminate or markedly reduce his or her drinking.

To elaborate on the cutoff of 28 drinks per week, clinically there are two reasons to be concerned about withdrawal symptoms. The prevention of morbidity and mortality is first and foremost, and it is our belief that the above criteria will adequately screen elderly patients for this danger. The second reason is less studied and may justify treating for withdrawal those patients who consume less than 28 drinks per week. One theory of early relapse posits the idea that withdrawal symptoms, even mild ones, place an individual at risk for relapse. If this is true, then aggressive treatment of withdrawal symptoms may improve clinical outcomes. We must emphasize that this is a hypothesis, so we are emphasizing the morbidity aspect in the algorithm.

It is also worth noting that this module is to be used and considered at any point during which the patient wants to quit or reduce his or her drinking, not just at the initial assessment.

Withdrawal Assessment

If the patient meets either of the above criteria, the clinician should conduct an interview to complete the Clinical Institute Withdrawal Assessment–Alcohol revised (CIWA–Ar) (Sullivan, Sykora, Schneiderman, & Naranjo, 1989). The CIWA–Ar is a well-validated assessment tool for determining the severity of alcohol withdrawal.

The total score on this initial CIWA–Ar will dictate the follow-up schedule (see altorithm at figure 5.1). If the CIWA–Ar score is below 8, the follow-up assessment can be by phone, if necessary. However, you are encouraged to see all patients in the office within 2 days. Each subsequent time you see the patient, you should complete a CIWA–Ar assessment and determine the steps for management of withdrawal symptoms until the patient is completely detoxified. At any point if the patient has two consecutive assessments in which the total score is below 8, the patient should be scheduled for his or her next routine appointment. You may want to call patients with whom you are using medication to alleviate symptoms on the days that you are not seeing them. This assessment is included as Appendix G.

Benzodiazepines are typically used to manage alcohol withdrawal. However, patients should be advised not to drink while taking a benzodiazepine such as oxazepam, and medical detoxification should only be considered for patients who are trying to become abstinent. These medicines alleviate symptoms and prevent their progression to a more serious state such as seizures. Benzodiazepines are cross-reactive with alcohol and essentially act to taper the effect of sudden drops in blood alcohol levels. The recommended medication for outpatient withdrawal management or detoxification is oxazepam (Serax). The metabolism of this medication is not affected by alcohol-related liver disease. Patients starting oxazepam should be given the information sheet for this medication, and symptoms that persist or worsen warrant an increase in total dosage until the symptoms have peaked. Once the withdrawal symptoms begin to lessen, the dosage should be tapered and discontinued by approximately 20% of the total dose per day or over the course of 4 to 7 days. It is also advisable to provide a higher dose of medication at night. Although the dose should be individualized, the following doses can be used as a guide for initiating treatment.

CIWA–Ar Total Score	Oxazepam dose
8–15	45–60 mg divided through the day
16–25	60–90 mg divided through the day

For CIWA–Ar scores over 25, clinicians are strongly encouraged to consider hospitalization. Other reasons for hospitalization may include failure of outpatient detoxification (continued drinking while on oxazepam or inability to reduce drinking); complex comorbid medical conditions likely to be affected by the use of benzodiazepines or caused by withdrawal such as severe obstructive pulmonary disease; patients with a coexisting seizure disorder or recent severe withdrawal symptoms; patients who are not likely to complete an outpatient detoxification such as severely demented individuals or persons unable to self-administer medications; or when outpatient medical detoxification is not available (e.g., when a physician is not available as part of the intervention).

CONCURRENT BENZODIAZEPINE OR OPIOID USE

The Problem

Historically benzodiazepines have been among the most commonly prescribed medications in the United States. The prevalence of benzodiazepine use increases with age, and older adults are more likely to take benzodiazepines chronically. Studies done in the 1970s and 1980s suggested that 10 to 15% of older adults were actively taking a benzodiazepine (Holroyd &

Duryee, 1997; Simon, VonKorff, Barlow, Pabiniak, & Wagner, 1996). In the last decade, however, serotonin-specific reuptake inhibitors (SSRIs) such as sertraline, paroxetine, and fluoxetine have been consistently among the most frequently prescribed medications in the U.S., and it is reasonable to speculate that the use of chronic benzodiazepines may have been supplanted by SSRIs.

Although there are reasons to hypothesize that benzodiazepine use may be less prevalent, benzodiazepine use among older adults, has been associated with falls, sleep disturbances, motor vehicle crashes, cognitive disturbances, and impairment in activities of daily living (ADLs) (Gales & Menard, 1995; Hemmelgarn, Suissa, Huang, Boivin, & Pinard, 1997; Herings, Stricker, deBoer, Bakker, & Sturmans, 1995; Newman, Enright, Manolio, Haponik, & Whal, 1997; Ried, Lohnson, & Gettman, 1998). Despite this literature, there is only one published study examining the benefits of withdrawing benzodiazepine (Habraken et al., 1997). In this study, 50 nursing home residents were randomly assigned to continue for 1 year on benzodiazepines or to be withdrawn and continue on a placebo. At both 6 and 12 months, the group receiving the placebo demonstrated improvement in ADLs. Previous research has also shown that benzodiazepines are often prescribed inappropriately for illnesses such as depression, psychosis, and chronic insomnia. Benzodiazepines can also be problematic for patients when combined with other psychoactive substances such as alcohol or antidepressants.

There are few, if any, protocols developed and tested for managing patients who have been taking benzodiazepines chronically and who need to be taken off these medications. Rickels and colleagues demonstrated that older adults could successfully be withdrawn from chronic benzodiazepine use, but they also showed that older patients are more apt to return to benzodiazepine use within three years of discontinuation (Rickels, Case, Schweizer, Garcia-Espana, & Fridman, 1991; Schweizer, Case, & Rickels, 1989). Thus, while there are clear risks associated with chronic benzodiazepine use, it is not entirely evident how best to screen for inappropriate use or to intervene in these patients.

Definition of Chronic Use

Although there is no universal definition for chronic benzodiazepine use and there is limited information regarding the risks and benefits of discontinuing benzodiazepines, the following definition is proposed by a consensus of the experts: Chronic benzodiazepine use is defined as the use of a benzodiazepine nearly every day for more than 3 months.

Withdrawal Procedure

For the purposes of this manual, chronic benzodiazepine use focuses only on individuals who also have significant alcohol consumption. However, it is advisable to consider a reduction in benzodiazepine as a goal for patients regardless of drinking status. After identifying patients who meet the criteria for chronic use, the clinician needs to discuss with the patient why he or she is on the medication, what the initial indication was for the medication, and whether the patient continues to derive benefit from the medication. At this point the clinician has to decide if there is sound justification for continuing the patient on the benzodiazepine. Cases that may justify continued chronic use may include a demonstrated effectiveness in reducing agitation associated with dementia, use in patients with terminal illnesses for comfort care, or use in patients with anxiety disorders that are refractory to other treatments such as SSRIs. Disorders that are not as justifiable include chronic insomnia, nervousness, depression, or chronic treatment of an alcohol use disorder.

Once the provider determines that there is limited justification for long-term use, the provider must make this recommendation to the patient. The provider's goal at this point is to educate the patient about the risks of long-term benzodiazepine use and the potential benefits of discontinuing the medication. The provider must also determine the presence of concurrent mental health issues such as depression or anxiety disorders, which will need to be successfully treated prior to discontinuing the benzodiazepines. If depression or anxiety symptoms are not treated, the probability of successfully discontinuing the benzodiazepine is markedly reduced. When managing patients who are drinking and using a benzodiazepine, we advise eliminating the alcohol use first, then addressing the benzodiazepine use.

Once the decision has been made to discontinue the benzodiazepine and all other mental health problems have been addressed, the medication can be slowly tapered. Based on the work of Schweizer and colleagues, the total dosage of benzodiazepine should be reduced by 25% per week (Schweizer et al., 1989). Therefore, the patient will receive 75% of the total dosage for 1 week, 50% of the total dosage for 1 week, and 25% of the total dosage the third week, followed by discontinuation. In other words, the medication will be stopped over the course of three weeks. During this time it is advisable to see the patient frequently, each week if possible, for support and encouragement.

HEAVY DRINKING

Heavy drinking among older adults is less common than at-risk or moderate drinking but may be overrepresented in certain populations such as those at addiction centers or Veterans Administration Medical Centers. Among older adults, heavy drinking is defined as more than 28 drinks per week or 3 or more days of binge drinking per week. The prevalence of heavy drinking is estimated to be 1% to 3% of the population with higher rates in clinical settings. Although heavy drinking is defined by quantity and frequency, persons who do drink in this range may very well also meet the diagnostic criteria for alcohol dependence. Despite the low prevalence, heavy drinking is associated with greater morbidity and mortality among older adults and may require a greater intensity of intervention in order to successfully reduce a patient's consumption. This module outlines some of the special concerns about patients who are heavy consumers and suggests further management strategies for these patients. Although this section of the manual focuses on heavy drinkers, some of these recommendations may apply to more moderate drinkers who have had difficulty managing their drinking with the brief intervention or who may have more morbidity associated with their moderate drinking.

Because brief interventions such as the ones described in this manual do not require a physician's involvement, it is important to consider the resources and limitations of the setting in which this program is being implemented. For example, in an addiction clinic where there will be a greater number of heavy drinkers, the clinic will need additional resources for the problems associated with heavy drinking, such as a physician to augment the brief intervention. In a primary care setting, if the intervention is being provided by a nurse or other nonphysician member of the team, the primary care physician may need guidance in managing the patient including reminders about which laboratory studies to order or how to manage withdrawal. Where there is no physician involvement, heavy drinkers may have to be referred to another setting.

Physical Health Concerns and Medical Evaluation

Heavy drinking and alcohol dependence can lead to a wide variety of physical health problems including liver disease, alcohol-related dementia, and cardiomyopathy. Heavy drinking and alcohol dependence can also exacerbate a number of physical health disorders such as cerebrovascular accidents (strokes), chronic obstructive lung disease, hypertension, and diabetes. Because of these relationships, it is particularly important that older heavy drinkers have a thorough physical examination with particular focus on the organ systems most likely to suffer alcohol-related damage.

In general the physical examination for a patient who is a heavy drinker would include a cognitive assessment and a focused neurologic examination for evidence of peripheral neuropathy and cranial nerve dysfunction. The clinician should also focus the examination on the liver, spleen, cardiovascular system, and on any evidence of trauma that may have occurred from falls or other accidents. In addition to recording blood pressure for signs of hypertension and weight for evidence of malnutrition, the following laboratory studies are recommended during an initial examination or annual follow-up:

- Complete blood count: Macrocytic anemia is often associated with heavy drinking.
- Liver studies (AST, ALT, and GGT): Elevations in any of these labs may be indicative of liver fibrosis or early liver failure. In patients who have abnormal elevations, especially GGT, the lab value can be used to track progress in treatment.

• Albumin: This is a marker of malnutrition and can be a sign of severe alcoholism.

Because people who are heavy drinkers tend also to have poor nutritional habits, it is common to recommend the addition of a multivitamin to their diets. Thiamine deficiency is a particular concern for heavy drinkers because it can lead to the neurologic disorder known as Wernicke—Korsakoff syndrome, whose principal features are dementia and psychotic symptoms. Therefore, it is also recommended that heavy drinkers be started on a thiamine supplement. The recommended dose is 100 mg per day and should be continued for a period of 3 months after the person has reduced or eliminated their drinking. Vitamins, and thiamine in particular, can be recommended for longer periods of time when patients continue to drink or when there is evidence of malnutrition or cognitive impairment.

Need for Detoxification

Heavier drinking increases the likelihood that a person will need a medical detoxification. This is especially true when the treatment goal calls for dramatically reducing or eliminating consumption. All patients who are heavy drinkers should be evaluated for their potential to experience withdrawal symptoms. Please refer to chapter 5 to learn more about managing this problem.

Adjunctive Treatments

Inpatient Detoxification and Rehabilitation

The availability of inpatient facilities has decreased dramatically over the last decade. Inpatient detoxification is warranted for patients with complex medical or psychiatric problems or for those who are unable to be detoxified successfully as an outpatient. It is vital to remember that detoxification is not a long-term solution for alcohol dependence and is merely an initial stop on the road to improved health. For a further discussion of when to refer for inpatient detoxification, see the detoxification section.

Inpatient rehabilitation and day treatment are potentially viable treatment options for patients who have not been successful on an outpatient basis. The dilemma here is that there are rarely age-specific programs available and cost may be an issue. Alternatives to formal treatments include senior centers, volunteer positions, and other activities that are structured and don't involve alcohol consumption.

Self-Help Groups

There are many different self-help groups available for patients with alcohol dependence. The most widely known is Alcoholics Anonymous. These groups can be extraordinarily helpful to some patients in providing a peer support network and a semistructured program to follow when trying to reduce drinking. If self-help groups are recommended for older adults, it is important that they include peers. Studies have demonstrated that older patients do significantly better in groups that include mostly peers than in mixed aged groups. Self-help groups also have traditionally focused on alcohol-dependent individuals and have set abstinence as the primary goal. Therefore, the at-risk drinker or non-alcohol-dependent drinker is likely to be put-off by the program. Because many self-help groups also incorporate a philosophy of a higher power, those who are apathetic about religion may find this unappealing. The bottom line here is that self-help groups are not for everyone and should not be a requirement of treatment especially in non-alcohol-dependent patients.

Pharmacotherapy

Pharmacotherapy of alcoholism should be reserved for patients with alcohol dependence. Currently there are two medications approved by the Food and Drug Administration for alcohol dependence: naltrexone and disulfiram. Because of potential life-threatening reactions when alcohol is mixed with disulfiram in patients who are medically ill, this medication is not recommended for use in older adults. Naltrexone, an opioid antagonist, has been shown to reduce the rate of relapse in both younger and older alcohol-dependent patients (Oslin, Liberto, O'Brien, Krois, & Norbeck, 1997). The exact mechanism is unknown, but the medication is thought to decrease the reward or pleasure associated with bingeing or heavy drinking. The medication is relatively well tolerated with the most common side effects being headache and nausea. There is a potential for liver toxicity in high doses, so the medication should not be used in patients with elevated total bilirubin levels. Naltrexone is given once daily in a dose of 50 mg, and it is recommended for all patients who are alcohol dependent and have struggled to achieve or maintain their treatment goals. While the duration of efficacy of naltrexone has only been established for 3 months, longer treatment durations have been used clinically and have been found to be useful for many patients.

Intensive Outpatient Programs

Intensive outpatient programs are often used during the early stages of recovery from alcohol dependence and typically involve 4– to 8–hour day programs 3 to 5 days a week. These programs often include psychoeducational programs, individual counseling, attendance at peer support groups, and vocational rehabilitation. Few of these programs have been developed specifically for older adults and may not focus on issues that are relevant to them. Programs with service of similar intensity include halfway houses, sheltered addiction programs and others that combine housing with addiction services. While these programs are typically geared toward younger and more severe patients, there may be a need to use these services and clinicians should be familiar with their availability.

While intensive specialized addiction programs may not be appropriate for patients with less severe problems, they do address one issue that is relevant to many older adults who may increase their drinking because of a lack of structured activities. Structured leisure time for older adults can be accomplished through intensive specialized addiction services and through volunteer activities, part-time employment, or participation in social organizations such as senior centers, churches, mosques, and fraternal organizations.

Group Therapy/Individual Psychotherapy

Group therapy with adjunctive individual therapy or counseling has been the mainstay of community-oriented addiction programs. Again, the services are structured predominately for younger adults, and many counselors and therapists have not received adequate training in issues related to older patients. In addition to staff training issues, research has suggested that placing older adults in groups with patients of all ages is not optimal to treatment outcomes. Older adults have better outcomes when placed in groups of other older adults with leaders who are knowledgeable about aging issues. In general these more formal services should be used for patients who do not respond to the brief interventions.

6

Resources

NATIONAL ORGANIZATIONS:

The National Institute on Alcohol Abuse and Alcoholism (NIAAA)
NIAAA
6000 Executive Boulevard
Bethesda, MD 20892–7003
(301)443–3860
http: /www.niaaa.nih.gov

Substance Abuse and Mental Health Services Administration
5600 Fishers Lane, Rockwall II
Rockville, MD 20857
(301)443-0365
http://www.samhsa.gov/

Center for Substance Abuse Prevention
5600 Fishers Lane, Rockwall II
Rockville, Maryland 20857
(301)443-0365
http://www.samhsa.gov/csap/index.htm

Center for Substance Abuse Treatment
5600 Fishers Lane, Rockwall II
Rockville, MD 20857
(301)443-0365
http://www.samhsa.gov/csat/csat.htm

Alcoholics Anonymous (AA)
Check the phonebook for a local chapter or write the national office at:
475 Riverside Drive, 11th fl.
New York, NY 10115
(212)870-3400

The National Council on Alcoholism and Drug Dependence, Inc. can refer you to treatment services in your area. Contact:

NCADD National Headquarters
12 West 21st Street 8th fl.
New York, NY 10010
(800)NCA-CALL (800-622-2255)

The National Institute on Aging offers a variety of resources on health and aging:

NIA Information Center
P.O. Box 8057
Gaithersburg, MD 20898-8057
(800)222-2225, TTY (800)222-4225
http://www.nia.nih.gov

PUBLISHED MATERIAL

Substance Abuse Among Older Adults, Treatment Improvement Protocol (TIP) Series 26.

Frederic C. Blow, PhD, Consensus Panel Chair
Substance Abuse and Mental Health Services Administration
Center for Substance Abuse Treatment
5600 Fishers Lane Rockwall II
Rockville, MD 20857
DHHS Publication No. (SMA) 98-3179
Printed 1998

Brief Interventions and Brief Therapies for Substance Abuse, Treatment Improvement Protocol (TIP) Series 34.

Kristen L Barry, PhD, Consensus Panel Chair
Substance Abuse and Mental Health Services Administration
Center for Substance Abuse Treatment
5600 Fishers Lane Rockwall II
Rockville, MD 20857
DHHS Publication No. (SMA) 99-3353
Printed 1999

Alcohol Problems and Aging.

E. S. L. Gomberg, A. M. Hegedus, R. A. Zucker, Eds.
NIAAA Research Monograph No. 33 NIH Pub No. 98-4163
Bethesda MD, NIAAA (1998)
Available free of cost by writing
NIAAA
P.O. Box 10686
Rockville, MD 20849-0686

Available on the web at: http://silk.nih.gov/silk/niaaa1/publication monograp.htm#online

Older Adults' Misuse of Alcohol, Medicines, and Other Drugs: Research and Practice Issues
   A. Gurnack, Ed. Springer Publishing Co., New York (1997)

Under the Rug: Substance Abuse and the Mature Woman
   Jeanne Reid
   June 1998

   The National Center on Addiction and Substance Abuse at Columbia University
   633 Third Avenue, 19th fl.
   New York, NY 10017-6706
   http://www.casacolumbia.org/publications1456/publications.htm

COMMUNITY SUBSTANCE-ABUSE RESOURCES

(Photocopy and complete for reference)

1. Community substance-abuse services:
Organization Name: _____
Phone _____
Hours _____
Contact person: _____ Insurance _____
Services available (circle):   counseling: alcohol/other drugs
       detox: alcohol/other drugs
       half-way house: men/women
       methadone program
       adolescent program/family program
       other: _____

2. Fee-for-service treatment programs:
Organization Name:_____
Phone _____
Hours _____ Contact person: _____
Type of facility (circle):
residential/outpatient/evening/adolescent/adult
Payment accepted: insurance/sliding scale/indigent care
Organization Name: _____
Phone _____
Hours _____ Contact person _____
Type of facility (circle):
residential/outpatient/evening/adolescent/adult
Payment accepted: insurance/sliding scale/indigent care

3. Individual therapist knowledgeable regarding substance abuse:
Name_____ Phone _____
Hours _____ Contact person _____
Type of facility (circle): residential/outpatient/evening/adolescent/adult
Payment accepted (circle all that apply): insurance/sliding scale/indigent
care
Name_____ Phone _____
Hours _____ Contact person _____
Type of facility (circle):
residential/outpatient/evening/adolescent/adult
Payment accepted (circle all that apply): insurance/sliding scale/indigent care

4. AA information number: _____

5. Al-Anon information number: _____

6. Narcotics Anonymous information number: _____

Appendix A

Health Promotion Workbook for Older Adults: Initial Session

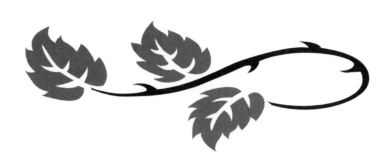

Health Promotion Workbook
For Older Adults:
Initial Session

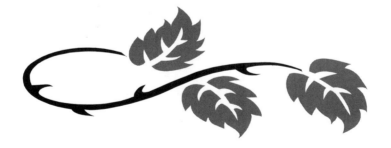

Today's date _____/_____/_____

PART 1: IDENTIFYING FUTURE GOALS

We will start by talking about some of your future goals. By that we mean, how would you like your life to improve and to be different in the future? It is often important to think about future goals when thinking about making changes in health habits.

What are some of your goals for the next 3 months to 1 year regarding your physical and emotional health?

_____

_____

_____

What are some of your goals for the next 3 months to 1 year regarding activities and hobbies?

_____

_____

_____

What are some of your goals for the next 3 months to 1 year regarding your relationships and social life?

_____

_____

_____

What are some of your goals in the next 3 months to 1 year regarding your financial situation or other parts of your life?

_____

_____

_____

PART 2: SUMMARY OF HEALTH HABITS

Let's review some of information about your health, behavior, or health habits.

EXERCISE

Days per week you participate in vigorous activity	□ none
	□ seldom
	□ 1–2 days per week
	□ 3–5 days per week
	□ 6–7 days per week
Minutes of exercise per day	□ not applicable
	□ less than 15 minutes
	□ 15–30 minutes
	□ more than 30 minutes

NUTRITION

Weight change in last 6 months	□ no change in weight
	□ gained more than 10 pounds
	□ lost more than 10 pounds
	□ don't know

TOBACCO USE

Tobacco used in last 6 months	□ no
	□ yes If yes, which ones?
	□ cigarettes
	□ chewing tobacco
	□ pipe
Average cigarettes smoked per day in the last 6 months	□ not applicable
	□ 1–9
	□ 10–19
	□ 20–29
	□ 30+

ALCOHOL USE

Drinking days per week	□ 1–2 days per week
	□ 3–4 days per week
	□ 5–6 days per week
	□ 7 days per week
Drinks per day	□ 1–2 drinks
	□ 3–4 drinks
	□ 5–6 drinks
	□ 7 or more

Binge drinking within last month   □ none
(four or more drinks/occasion for   □ 1–2 binges
women; four or more drinks/occasion   □ 3–5 binges
for men)   □ 6–7 binges
                                          □ 8 or more

On days that you do not drink do you   □ No
feel anxious, have greater difficulty   □ Yes
sleeping than usual, feel your heart
racing, have heart palpitations, or have
the shakes or hand tremors?

Are there any of these health behaviors (exercise, nutrition, tobacco use, alcohol use) with which you would like some help?

□ No   □ Yes   If yes, which ones?
                                     □ exercise
                                     □ nutrition
                                     □ tobacco use
                                     □ alcohol usee

PART 3: STANDARD DRINKS

The drinks shown below, in normal measure, contain roughly the same amount of pure alcohol. You can think of each one as a *standard drink.*

What is a standard drink?
One standard drink =

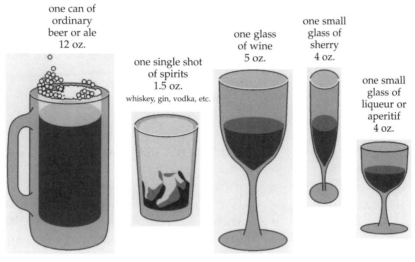

one can of
ordinary
beer or ale
12 oz.

one single shot
of spirits
1.5 oz.
whiskey, gin, vodka, etc.

one glass
of wine
5 oz.

one small
glass of
sherry
4 oz.

one small
glass of
liqueur or
aperitif
4 oz.

PART 4: TYPES OF OLDER DRINKERS IN THE U.S. POPULATION

It is helpful to think about the amount of alcohol consumed by older adults in the United States and by you. There are different types of drinkers among the older adult population, and these types can be explained by different patterns of alcohol consumption. These include:

<u>Types</u>	<u>Patterns of alcohol consumption</u>
Abstainers and light drinkers	• drink no alcohol or less than three drinks per month • alcohol use does not affect health or result in negative consequences
Moderate drinkers	• drink three or fewer times per week • drink one or two standard drinks per occasion • alcohol use does not affect health or result in negative consequences • at times moderate drinkers consume NO alcohol, such as before driving or while operating machinery
At-risk drinkers	• drink more than seven standard drinks per week • at risk for negative health and social consequences
Alcohol abuse or dependence	• heavy drinking has led to a physical need for alcohol and to other problems

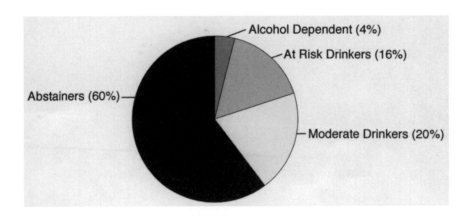

PART 5: CONSEQUENCES OF AT-RISK OR PROBLEM DRINKING

Drinking alcohol can affect your *physical health, emotional and social well being, and relationships.*

The following are some of the positive effects that people sometimes describe as a result of drinking alcohol. Let's place a check mark by the ones that you feel apply to you.

☐ Temporary high ☐ Relaxation   ☐ Avoid uncomfortable feelings

☐ Forget problems ☐ Sense of confidence   ☐ Ease in speaking one's mind

☐ Enjoy the taste   ☐ Temporary lower stress   ☐ Social ease

The following are some of the *negative consequences* that may result from drinking. Let's place a check mark by any of these problems that are affecting you regardless of whether you believe they are related to your drinking.

☐ Difficulty coping with stressful situations   ☐ Sleep problems   ☐ Accidents/falls

☐ Depression   ☐ Memory problems or   ☐ Relationship problems confusion

☐ Loss of independence   ☐ Malnutrition   ☐ Increased risk of assault

☐ Problems in community activities   ☐ Reduced effectiveness   ☐ Financial problems of medications

☐ High blood pressure   ☐ Increased side effects from medication   ☐ Stomach pain

☐ Sexual performance problems   ☐ Liver problems

PART 6: REASONS TO QUIT OR CUT DOWN ON YOUR DRINKING

The purpose of this step is to think about the best reason for you to quit or cut down on your drinking. The reasons will be different for different people.

The following list identifies some of the reasons for which people decide to cut down or quit drinking. Put an X in the box by the three most important reasons that YOU want to quit or cut down on your drinking. Perhaps you can think of other reasons that are not on this list.

☐ To consume fewer empty calories (alcoholic drinks contain many calories)
☐ To sleep better
☐ To maintain independence
☐ To feel better
☐ To save money
☐ To be happier
☐ To reduce the possibility that I will be injured in a car crash
☐ To have better family relationships
☐ To participate more in community activities
☐ To have better friendships
☐ Other: _____

Write down the three most important reasons you choose to cut down or quit drinking.

1. _____

2. _____

3. _____

Think about the consequences of continuing to drink heavily. Now think about how your life might improve if you decide to change your drinking habits by cutting down or quitting. What improvements do you anticipate?

Physical health:

Mental health:

Family:

Other relationships:

Activities:

PART 7: DRINKING AGREEMENT

The purpose of this step is to decide on a drinking limit for yourself for a particular period of time. Negotiate with your health care provider so you can both agree on a reasonable goal. A reasonable goal for some people is abstinence, that is, not drinking any alcohol.

As you develop this agreement, answer the following questions:
- How many standard drinks?
- How frequently?
- For what period of time?

DRINKING AGREEMENT
Date _____
Patient's signature _____
Clinician's signature _____

DRINKING DIARY CARD

One way to keep track of how much you drink is the use of drinking diary cards. One card is used for each week. Every day record the number of drinks you had. At the end of the week add up the total number of drinks you had during the week.

DIARY CARD

KEEP TRACK OF WHAT YOU DRINK OVER THE NEXT 7 DAYS

STARTING DATE _____

	Beer	Wine	Liquor	Number
Sunday				
Monday				
Tuesday				
Wednesday				
Thursday				
Friday				
Saturday				
			Week's total:	

KEEP TRACK OF WHAT YOU DRINK OVER THE NEXT 7 DAYS

STARTING DATE _____

	Beer	Wine	Liquor	Number
Sunday				
Monday				
Tuesday				
Wednesday				
Thursday				
Friday				
Saturday				
			Week's total:	

PART 8: HANDLING RISKY SITUATIONS

Your desire to drink may change according to your mood, the people you are with, and the availability of alcohol. Think about your last periods of drinking.

Here are examples of risky situations. The following list may help you remember situations that can result in at-risk drinking.

- social get-togethers
- boredom
- tension
- feeling lonely
- feelings of failure
- frustration
- use of tobacco

- sleeplessness
- family
- friends
- criticism
- dinner parties
- children and grandchildren
- TV or magazine ads

- anger
- watching television
- other people drinking
- certain places
- after regular daily activities
- weekends
- arguments

What are the situations that make you want to drink at a risky level. Please write them down.

1. _____

2. _____

Ways to Cope With Risky Situations

It is important to figure out how you can make sure you will not go over drinking limits when you are tempted. Here are examples:

- Telephone a friend
- Go for a walk

- Call on a neighbor
- Watch a movie

- Read a book
- Participate in an activity you like

Some of these ideas may not work for you, but other methods of dealing with risky situations may work. Identify ways you could cope with the specific risky situations you listed above.

1. For the first risky situation or feeling, write down different ways of coping.

_____

_____

2. For the second risky situation or feeling, write down different ways of coping.

_____

_____

Think about other situations and ways you could cope without using alcohol.

PART 9: VISIT SUMMARY

We've covered a great deal of information today. Changing your behavior, especially drinking patterns, can be a difficult challenge. The following pointers may help you stick with your new behavior and maintain the drinking limit agreement, especially during the first few weeks when it is most difficult. Remember that you are changing a habit, and that it can be hard work. It becomes easier with time.

- Remember your drinking limit goal: _____
- Read this workbook frequently.
- Congratulate yourself every time you are tempted to drink above limits and are able to resist, because you are breaking an old habit.
- Whenever you feel very uncomfortable, tell yourself that the feeling will pass.
- At the end of each week, think about how many days you have been abstinent (consumed no alcohol) or have been a light or moderate drinker.
- Some people have days during which they drink too much. If that happens to you, DON'T GIVE UP. Just start again the next day.
- You should always feel welcome to call your primary care provider for assistance or in case of an emergency.

THANKS FOR TRYING THIS PROGRAM.

Please bring your drinking diary cards to your next visit to review with the nurse or your physician.

Appendix B

Health Promotion Workbook for Older Adults: Follow-up Session

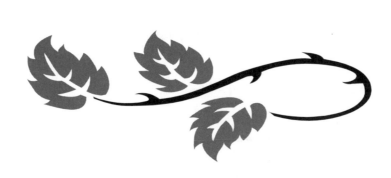

Health Promotion Workbook:
For Older Adults
Follow-up Session

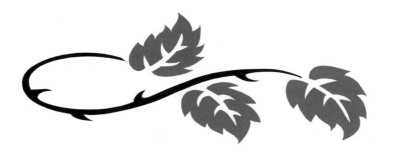

Today's Date _____ / _____ / _____

PART 1: PURPOSE OF TODAY'S VISIT

At your initial visit we discussed how alcohol use can affect your overall health and well-being. At the conclusion of that visit you signed a drinking agreement and agreed that we could meet again to further discuss you alcohol use.

Today we will review how much you have been drinking since our last visit and work to renew or revise your drinking goal.

PART 2: REVIEW OF ALCOHOL USE

Let's start by reviewing your drinking diary cards from your last visit.

If you do not have them or were unable to complete them then let's proceed on.

Now let's review your drinking over the last week.

WHAT DID YOU DRINK OVER THE LAST SEVEN DAYS?

STARTING DATE _____

	Beer	Wine	Liquor	Number
Sunday				
Monday				
Tuesday				
Wednesday				
Thursday				
Friday				
Saturday				
			Week's total:	

PART 3: REVIEW OF CHANGES IN ALCOHOL USE

According to your drinking diary, your
  alcohol use

☐ decreased
☐ stayed the same
☐ increased

Did you meet your goal that you had set at
  our last meeting?

☐ No
☐ Yes

Now let's talk about the days that you tried to cut down or not
drink, even if you were unable to cut down or stop. Tell me
about the times you tried or succeeded in cutting down or stopping your drinking. Note below the times that you attempted
or quite drinking.

1. _____

_____

2. _____

_____

3. _____

_____

Did you find it difficult to try to cut down on your
  drinking? If so what was difficult?

☐ No
☐ Yes

1. _____

2. _____

3. _____

If you cut down, were there positive aspects to
  reducing your drinking?
If so what were the positive things?

☐ No
☐ Yes

1. _____

2. _____

3. _____

PART 4: CONSEQUENCES OF AT-RISK OR PROBLEM DRINKING

As we discussed at our last visit, drinking alcohol can affect your *physical health, emotional and social well being, and relationships.*

Let's review some of the positive effects that people sometimes describe as a result of drinking alcohol. Let's place a check mark by the ones that you feel still apply to you.

□ Temporary high	□ Relaxation	□ Avoid uncomfortable feelings
□ Forget problems	□ Sense of confidence	□ Ease in speaking one's mind
□ Enjoy the taste	□ Temporary lower stress	
□ Social ease		

If you changed your drinking, have you noticed a change for the better or worse in any of these areas? If you reduced your drinking have you missed any of these effects?

The following are some of the *negative consequences* that may result from drinking. Let's place a check mark by any of these problems that are continuing to affect you regardless of whether you believe they are related to your drinking.

□ Difficulty coping with stressful situations	□ Sleep problems	□ Accidents/falls
□ Depression	□ Memory problems or confusion	□ Relationship problems
□ Loss of independence	□ Malnutrition	□ Increased risk of assault
□ Problems in community activities	□ Reduced effectiveness of medications	□ Financial problems
□ High blood pressure	□ Increased side effects	□ Stomach pain
□ Sexual performance problems		□ Liver problems

Have any of these areas gotten better or worse since our last visit? Did changing your drinking affect any of these areas?

PART 5: REASONS TO QUIT OR CUT DOWN ON YOUR DRINKING

Let's review the reasons you identified for reducing or quitting your drinking. First let's mark the areas that were the most important reasons YOU wanted to quit or cut down on your drinking from the first time we met. Have any of these changed? Which ones would you mark at this time?

	Previous Selections	Current Reasons
To consume fewer empty calories		
(alcoholic drinks contain many calories)	☐	☐
To sleep better	☐	☐
To maintain independence	☐	☐
To feel better	☐	☐
To save money	☐	☐
To be happier	☐	☐
To reduce the possibility that I will be		
injured in a car crash	☐	☐
To have better family relationships	☐	☐
To participate more in community activities	☐	☐
To have better friendships	☐	☐
To improve my health	☐	☐
Other: _____	☐	☐

PART 6: DRINKING AGREEMENT

We want to review your decision to reduce your drinking and decide on a drinking limit for yourself. Negotiate with your health care provider so you can both agree on a reasonable goal. A reasonable goal for some people is abstinence, that is not drinking any alcohol.

As you develop this agreement, answer the following questions:

- How many standard drinks (see below)?
- How frequently?
- For what period of time?

DRINKING AGREEMENT

Date _____

Patient's signature _____

Clinician's signature _____

The drinks shown below, in normal measure, contain roughly the same amount of pure alcohol. You can think of each one as a *standard drink*.

What is a standard drink?
One standard drink =

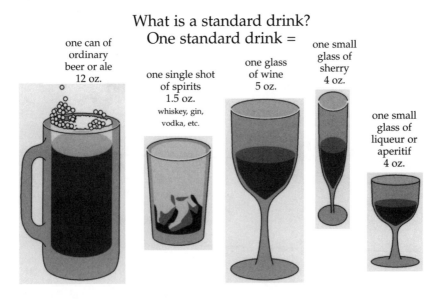

one can of ordinary beer or ale 12 oz.

one single shot of spirits 1.5 oz. whiskey, gin, vodka, etc.

one glass of wine 5 oz.

one small glass of sherry 4 oz.

one small glass of liqueur or aperitif 4 oz.

PART 7: WAYS TO COPE WITH RISKY SITUATIONS

It is important to find ways to make sure you will not go over drinking limits when you are tempted. Here are examples:

- Telephone a friend
- Call on a neighbor
- Read a book
- Go for a walk
- Watch a movie
- Participate in an activity or hobby you like

Some of these ideas may not work for you, but other methods of dealing with risky situations may work. Identify ways you could cope with the specific risky situations.

What ways did you try already? Did these work or not? Why?

1. _____

_____

2. _____

_____

3. _____

_____

What are some of the things you want to try or continue doing in order to help reduce your drinking further or to maintain the goal that you have achieved?

1. _____

_____

2. _____

_____

3. _____

_____

Think about other situations and ways you could cope without using alcohol.

PART 8: VISIT SUMMARY

We've covered a great deal of information today. Changing your behavior, especially drinking patterns, can be a difficult challenge. The following pointers may help you stick with your new behavior and maintain the drinking limit agreement, especially during the first few weeks when it is most difficult. Remember that you are changing a habit, and that it can be hard work. It becomes easier with time.

- Remember your drinking limit goal: _____
- Read this workbook and your first workbook frequently.
- Congratulate yourself every time you are tempted to drink above limits and are able to resist, because you are breaking an old habit.
- Whenever you feel very uncomfortable, tell yourself that the feeling will pass.
- At the end of each week, think about how many days you have been abstinent (consumed no alcohol) or have been a light or moderate drinker.
- Some people have days during which they drink too much. If that happens to you, DON'T GIVE UP. Just start again the next day.
- You should always feel welcome to call your primary care provider for assistance or in case of an emergency.

THANKS FOR TRYING THIS PROGRAM.

Please bring your drinking diary cards to your next visit to review with the nurse or your physician.

Appendix C

Drinking Cards

DRINKING DIARY CARD

We would like you to continue to keep track of how much you drink using the drinking diary cards. One card is used for each week. Every day record the number of drinks you had. At the end of the week add up the total number of drinks you had during the week.

DIARY CARD

KEEP TRACK OF WHAT YOU DRINK OVER THE NEXT 7 DAYS

STARTING DATE _____

	Beer	Wine	Liquor	Number
Sunday				
Monday				
Tuesday				
Wednesday				
Thursday				
Friday				
Saturday				
			Week's total:	

KEEP TRACK OF WHAT YOU DRINK OVER THE NEXT 7 DAYS

STARTING DATE _____

	Beer	Wine	Liquor	Number
Sunday				
Monday				
Tuesday				
Wednesday				
Thursday				
Friday				
Saturday				
			Week's total:	

KEEP TRACK OF WHAT YOU DRINK OVER THE NEXT 7 DAYS

STARTING DATE _____

	Beer	Wine	Liquor	Number
Sunday				
Monday				
Tuesday				
Wednesday				
Thursday				
Friday				
Saturday				
			Week's total:	

KEEP TRACK OF WHAT YOU DRINK OVER THE NEXT 7 DAYS

STARTING DATE _____

	Beer	Wine	Liquor	Number
Sunday				
Monday				
Tuesday				
Wednesday				
Thursday				
Friday				
Saturday				
			Week's total:	

DRINKING DIARY CARD

One way to keep track of how much you drink is by the use of drinking diary cards. One card is used for each week. Every day record the number of drinks you had. At the end of the week add up the total number of drinks you had during the week.

DIARY CARD

KEEP TRACK OF WHAT YOU DRINK OVER THE NEXT 7 DAYS

STARTING DATE _____

	Beer	Wine	Liquor	Number
Sunday				
Monday				
Tuesday				
Wednesday				
Thursday				
Friday				
Saturday				
			Week's total:	

KEEP TRACK OF WHAT YOU DRINK OVER THE NEXT 7 DAYS

STARTING DATE _____

	Beer	Wine	Liquor	Number
Sunday				
Monday				
Tuesday				
Wednesday				
Thursday				
Friday				
Saturday				
			Week's total:	

Appendix D

Patient Educational Handout

This handout is intended for use in waiting rooms, as handouts to patients whom you might be concerned about, for health fairs, or for any other applicable use. It is formatted to fit on the back and front of one third of a standard 8.5" x 11" sheet of stock of paper. Heavier card stock with a soft color is suggested. You are encouraged to redesign it to include additional information such as local phone numbers, to add logos, or to resize it to fit a different presentation format. The material can be copied for clinical use but is otherwise copyrighted.

Healthy Alcohol Use for Older Adults
(65 and over)

Recommended Drinking Limits

- **No more than 1 drink a day for people over 65.**

- **No more than 2 drinks on any given day.**

- **No drinking for people with past problems of alcoholism or who have chronic illnesses (such as diabetes, emphysema, Alzheimer's disease, or depression).**

- **No drinking while taking certain medications.**

Why should older adults drink less than younger adults? Physical changes associated with aging make older adults more vulnerable to the effects of alcohol. Two drinks for an older adult is like three in younger adults.

Standard Drinks

Beer, wine, mixed drinks, and hard liquor all contain equal amounts of alcohol.

Risks of Alcohol Use
- Heart problems
- Strokes by bleeding
- Falls and fractures
- Adverse reactions with other medications
- Impaired driving
- Memory problems
- Sleep problems
- Stomach problems
- Liver problems

Possible benefits when consumption is within the recommended level
- Decreased risk of heart disease
- Decreased risk of stroke by blockage
- Easier to socialize

Older adults should consider the possible problems and benefits of alcohol use for themselves if they are thinking of having more than 1 drink a day.

For more information call 215-615-3083

Appendix E

Typical Screening, Assessment, and Follow-up Instruments

TYPICAL SCREENING QUESTIONS

1. Now I would like to ask you
   some questions about your use of
   alcoholic beverages such as beer,
   wine, wine coolers, or hard liquor
   such as vodka, gin, or whiskey.
   Have you had a drink of alcohol
   in the past year? (If the person is
   unable to answer, or refuses to
   answer this portion of the   No (interview ends)...0
   interview ends.)   Yes (continue with #2)...1

2. During the last 3 months, how many
   days per week on average would you have
   had an alcoholic beverage? *(answers range
   from 0 to 7 only)*   _____

3. During the last 3 months, how many drinks on
   average would you have consumed on a day
   that you drink?   _____

4. On days that you drank any alcohol during the
   last 3 months, how many times did you drink
   four or more drinks in one day?   _____

Note: A single mixed drink   = 1 drink
        A 12 oz. Beer   = 1 drink
        A shot of hard liquor   = 1 drink
        A pint of hard liquor   = 11 drinks
        A fifth of hard liquor = 18 drinks
        A 4 oz. glass of wine   = 1 drink
        A pint of wine   = 5 drinks
        A bottle of wine (40 oz.) = 8 drinks

*This screen will be considered positive if a patient exceeds seven drinks
per week (determined by multiplying the response to question #2 to
the response to question #3). The screen will also be considered positive if the patient has had more than two binge episodes in the prior 3
months (response to question #4 > 2). A positive screen indicates the
need to proceed with a more in-depth assessment of patient's drinking
and possible alcohol-related problems.*

ASSESSMENT AND FOLLOW-UP QUESTIONS

1. I would like to ask some questions   No (interview ends)...0
   about your use of alcoholic   Yes (continue with #2)...1
   beverages such as beer, wine, wine
   coolers, or hard liquor such as
   vodka, gin, or whiskey. Have you
   had a drink of alcohol in the past
   year? (If the person is unable to
   answer or refuses to answer, this
   portion of the interview ends)

2. During the last week, did you have   No (continue with #4)...0
   any drink containing alcohol?   Yes (continue with #3)...1

3. I would like to know the number
   of alcoholic drinks you've had
   each day in the last week.
   Today is _____. Let's
   begin with yesterday.
   How many drinks of beer, wine,
   or liquor did you have on (Name
   day of week)?

	Sunday	Monday	Tuesday	Wednesday	Thursday	Friday	Saturday	Total
Number of drinks	____	____	____	____	____	____	____	____

Fill in the number of drinks consumed on each of the 7 days prior to the interview. The total represents the total number of drinks per week.

Note: A single mixed drink   =   1 drink
        A 12 oz. beer   =   1 drink
        A shot of hard liquor   =   1 drink
        A pint of hard liquor   =   11 drinks
        A fifth of hard liquor   =   18 drinks
        A 4 oz. glass of wine   =   1 drink
        A pint of wine   =   3+ drinks
        A bottle of wine (40 oz.) = 8 drinks

4. During the last 3 months, on days that you drank
   any alcohol, how many times did you drink four
   or more drinks in one day?   _____

SCREENING QUESTIONS FOR OPIOID OR BENZODIAZEPINE USE

Are you currently taking any of the following medications: Valium (diazepam), Xanax (alprazolam), Ativan (lorazepam), Demerol (chlordiazepoxide), Klonopin (clonazepam), Tranxene (clorazepate), ProSom (estazolam), Serax (oxazepam), Dalmane (flurazepam), or Restoril (temazepam)?

No ... 0
Yes ... 1

If yes, circle the name of the medication most commonly used.

On average how many days per week will you take one of these medications? _____

How many months have you been taking these medications? _____

What is the usual dose that you take? ___mg or pills
circle mg or pills

Are you currently taking any of the following medications: products containing codeine such as Percocet, Percodan, Tylenol #3, or other medications such as Demerol (mederidine) or Darvon (poxyphene)?

No ... 0
Yes ... 1

If yes, circle the name of the medication most commonly used.

On average how many days per week will you take one of these medications? _____

How many months have you been taking these medications? _____

Appendix F

Short Michigan Alcohol Screening Test: Geriatric version (SMAST–G)

SMAST–G

	YES	NO
In the past year:		
1. When talking with others, do you ever underestimate how much you actually drink?	(1)	(0)
2. After a few drinks, have you sometimes not eaten or been able to skip a meal because you didn't feel hungry?	(1)	(0)
3. Does having a few drinks help decrease your shakiness or tremors?	(1)	(0)
4. Does alcohol sometimes make it hard for you to remember parts of the day or night?	(1)	(0)
In the past year:		
5. Do you usually take a drink to relax or calm your nerves?	(1)	(0)
6. Do you drink to take your mind off your problems?	(1)	(0)
7. Have you ever increased your drinking after experiencing a loss in your life?	(1)	(0)
8. Has a doctor or nurse ever said they were worried or concerned about your drinking?	(1)	(0)
9. Have you ever made rules to manage your drinking?	(1)	(0)
10. When you feel lonely, does having a drink help?	(1)	(0)

Total SMAST–G Score (0–10) _____

Appendix G

Clinical Institute Withdrawal Assessment for Alcohol (CIWA–Ar)

CLINICAL INSTITUTE WITHDRAWAL
ASSESSMENT FOR ALCOHOL (CIWA–AR)

Date (month/day)			
1. TREMOR: (*Assess with arms extended and fingers apart*) 0 = no tremor 1 = tremor not visibly apparent, can be felt by placing fingertips lightly against patient's fingertips 4 = tremor is moderate 7 = marked tremor even when arms are not extended			
2. PAROXYSMAL SWEATS: (*At time of observation*) 0 = no sweat visible 1 = barely perceptible sweating, palms moist 4 = beads of sweat obviously observable on forehead 7 = drenching sweats			
3. CLOUDING OF SENSORIUM: (*At time of observation*) 0 = no evidence of clouding of sensorium 1 = cannot do serial 7 subtractions or is uncertain about date 2 = disoriented for date by no more than 2 calendar days 3 = disoriented for date by more than 2 calendar days 4 = disoriented for place and/or person			
4. AGITATION / RESTLESSNESS: (*Based on present movement. Do not confuse with anxiety or tremor*) 0 = normal activity 1 = somewhat more than normal activity 4 = moderately fidgety and restless 7 = paces back and forth during most of the interview, or thrashes about constantly			
5. PULSE: (*At time of observation*) 0 = 89 or below 4 = 105–109 1 = 90–94 5 = 110–114 2 = 95–99 6 = 115–119 3 = 100–104 7 = 120 or higher			
6. NAUSEA & VOMITING: (*Ask, "Do you feel sick to your stomach? Have you vomited?" Observation.*) 0 = no nausea and no vomiting 1 = mild nausea with no vomiting 4 = intermittent nausea with dry heaves 7 = constant nausea, frequent dry heaves, and vomiting			

7. ANXIETY: (*Ask, "Do you feel nervous?" Observation.*)			
0 = no anxiety, at ease 1 = mildly anxious 4 = moderately anxious, or guarded, so anxiety is inferred 7 = equivalent to acute panic states as seen in severe delirium or acute schizophrenic reactions			
8. TACTILE DISTURBANCES: (*Ask "Have you any itching, pins-and-needles sensations, burning, or numbness or do you feel bugs crawling on or under your skin?" Observation.*) 0 = none 1 = very mild itching, pins and needles, burning or numbness 2 = mild itching, pins and needles, burning or numbness 4 = moderately severe hallucinations 5 = severe hallucinations 6 = extremely severe hallucinations 7 = continuous hallucinations			
9. AUDITORY DISTURBANCES: (*Ask "Are you more aware of sounds around you? Are they harsh? Do they frighten you? Are you hearing things you know are not there?" Observation.*) 0 = not present 1 = very mild harshness or ability to frighten 2 = mild harshness or ability to frighten 3 = moderate harshness or ability to frighten 4 = moderately severe hallucinations 5 = severe hallucinations 6 = extremely severe hallucinations 7 = continuous hallucinations			
10. VISUAL DISTURBANCES: (*Ask "Does the light appear to be too bright? Does it hurt your eyes? Are you seeing anything that is disturbing to you? Are you seeing things you know are not there?" Observation.*) 0 = not present 1 = very mild sensitivity 2 = mild sensitivity 3 = moderate sensitivity 4 = moderately severe hallucinations 5 = severe hallucinations 6 = extremely severe hallucinations 7 = continuous hallucinations			

11. HEADACHE, FULLNESS IN HEAD: (*Ask "Does
your head feel different?" "Does it feel like there is a
band around your head?" Do not rate for dizziness or
lightheadedness. Otherwise, rate severity.*)
0 = not present
1 = very mild
2 = mild
3 = moderate
4 = moderately severe
5 = severe
6 = very severe
7 = extremely severe
Total score
Interviewer's initials

Appendix H

Oxazepam Education Form

OXAZEPAM EDUCATION FORM

Detoxification

The definition of detoxification, or "detox," is a medically supervised and safe way to rid the body of alcohol or drugs. Detox is the first step toward substance abuse treatment and a successful program of recovery.

Withdrawal

People addicted to drugs, alcohol, or cigarettes may experience withdrawal when the substance is stopped. Proper medical care can prevent serious mental or physical reactions. "Withdrawal" symptoms can range anywhere from sleep problems, shakes, tremors, and depression to seizures or death.

Medication

Oxazepam is used to treat and prevent the worsening of alcohol withdrawal. As your body returns to normal, your health care provider will slowly decrease your dose of oxazepam. It is important to remember not to mix oxazepam with alcohol or other drugs. Mixing oxazepam with alcohol can be dangerous enough to result in serious health problems.

General Guidelines

Read and follow the individual directions on your oxazepam prescription as prescribed by your health care provider. If you feel drowsy or slowed down or if your speech slurs, increase the amount of time between doses. If slurred speech continues, stop taking your medication and contact your physician's office. If you feel shaky, nauseous, restless, nervous, or anxious 1 hour after taking your regularly scheduled medication, contact your physician's office. Call if these symptoms do not improve, or if you have a temperature of more than 100°F, or if nausea or vomiting prevent keeping medication down.
- Avoid alcohol.
- Rest your body and give it an opportunity to heal.
- Drink 6–8 glasses of nonalcoholic, decaffeinated fluids daily.
- Eat healthy meals.
- Use caution when driving or working with heavy machinery.

Contact

If you have any further questions about this medication or experience side effects, contact your physician's office at _____.

Conclusion

I verify that I have read this form and understand the above information. I agree not to consume alcohol during treatment with oxazepam.

_____ _____ _____

Signature of Patient   Healthcare Provider   Date

Appendix I

Health Promotion Workbook: Initial Session Spanish Version

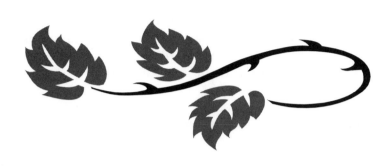

Health Promotion Workbook
For Older Adults:
Initial Session—Spanish
Version

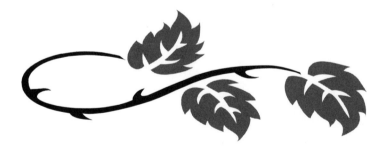

Fecha de hoy ___ / ___ / ___

1ª PARTE: IDENTIFICACION DE SUS METAS FUTURAS

Vamos a comenzar hablando de algunas de sus metas futuras. Es decir, ¿cómo le gustaría que su vida mejorara o fuera diferente en el futuro? A menudo, es importante pensar en metas futuras cuando se piensa cambiar los hábitos de salud.

¿Cuáles son algunas de sus metas para los próximos 3 meses a 1 año en términos de su salud física y emocional?

_____

_____

_____

¿Cuáles son algunas de sus metas para los próximos 3 meses a 1 año en términos de actividades y pasatiempos?

_____

_____

_____

¿Cuáles son algunas de sus metas para los próximos 3 meses a 1 año en términos de sus relaciones y vida personal?

_____

_____

_____

¿Cuáles son algunas de sus metas para los próximos 3 meses a 1 año en términos de su situación financiera u otros aspectos de su vida?

_____

_____

_____

2ª PARTE: RESUMEN DE LOS HABITOS DE SALUD

Vamos a revisar la información sobre su salud, comportamiento y hábitos de salud.

EJERCICIO

Número de días por semana que participa usted en actividades vigorosas:

☐ Ninguno
☐ Raramente
☐ 1–2 días por semana
☐ 3–5 días por semana
☐ 6–7 días por semana

Minutos de ejercicio que hace por día:

☐ No aplica
☐ Menos de 15 minutos
☐ 15–30 minutos
☐ Más de 30 minutos

NUTRICION

Cambios de peso en los últimos seis meses:

☐ No ha cambiado de peso
☐ Ha engordado más de 10 libras
☐ Ha perdido más de 10 libras
☐ No sabe

USO DE TABACO

Uso de tabaco en los últimos seis meses:

☐ No
☐ Sí ¿Qué usa?
    ☐ Cigarrillos
    ☐ Tabaco masticable
    ☐ Pipa

Promedio de cigarrillos que ha fumado por día en los últimos seis meses:

☐ No aplica
☐ 1–9
☐ 10–19
☐ 20–29
☐ 30+

CONSUMO DE ALCOHOL

Número de días en que consume   ☐ 1–2 días por semana
alcohol por semana: ☐ 3–4 días por semana
                                       ☐ 5–6 días por semana
                                       ☐ 7 días por semana

Número de bebidas alcohólicas por día: ☐ 1–2 bebidas
                                       ☐ 3–4 bebidas
                                       ☐ 5–6 bebidas
                                       ☐ 7 o más

Veces en que consumió en exceso en
el último mes: (cuatro bebidas   ☐ Ninguna
alcohólicas o más/ocasión para las   ☐ 1–2 veces
mujeres; cuatro bebidas alcohólicas   ☐ 3–5 veces
o más/ocasión para los hombres)   ☐ 6–7 veces
                                       ☐ 8 veces o más

En los días en que no toma alcohol, ¿se   ☐ No
siente usted ansioso/a, tiene más   ☐ Sí
dificultad de lo normal para dormir,
tiene taquicardia o palpitaciones, o
tiene sacudidas o temblores de mano?

Le gustaría recibir ayuda con alguno de estos hábitos de salud? (el
ejercicio, la nutrición, el uso de tabaco o cigarrillos, o el uso de
alcohol)
☐ No   ☐ Sí   De ser así, con cuales?
                                       ☐ El ejercicio
                                       ☐ La nutrición
                                       ☐ El uso de tabaco
                                       ☐ El uso de alcohol

3ª PARTE: BEBIDAS ESTANDARES

Las bebidas que aparecen a continuación, en tamaño normal, contienen básicamente la misma cantidad de alcohol puro. Se puede pensar en cada una como una bebida estándar.

¿Que constituye una bebida estándar?
un bebida estándar equivale =

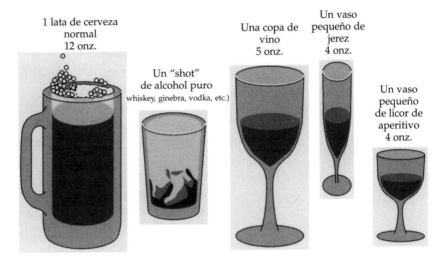

1 lata de cerveza
normal
12 onz.

Un "shot"
de alcohol puro
whiskey, ginebra, vodka, etc.)

Una copa de
vino
5 onz.

Un vaso
pequeño de
jerez
4 onz.

Un vaso
pequeño
de licor de
aperitivo
4 onz.

4ª PARTE: TIPOS DE PERSONAS MAYORES QUE TOMAN ALCOHOL EN LA POBLACION DE LOS E.E.U.U.

Conviene pensar en la cantidad de alcohol que consumen las personas mayores en los Estados Unidos así como la cantidad que toma usted. Existen diferentes tipos de bebedores entre la población de personas mayores, y se pueden explicar con diferentes patrones en el consumo de alcohol. Estos incluyen:

Tipo:	Patrones de consumo de alcohol:
Abstemios y personas	• No tomar alcohol o tomar menos de tres tragos por mes
que beben muy poco	• El uso de alcohol no afecta su salud ni tiene consecuencias negativas
Bebedores moderados	• Tomar alcohol tres veces o menos por semana
	• Tomar una o dos bebidas estándares por ocasión
	• El uso de alcohol no afecta la salud ni tiene consecuencias negativas
	• Los bebedores moderados NO consumen alcohol en ciertos momentos como antes de conducir o mientras operan una máquina etc.
Bebedores en riesgo	• Tomar más de siete bebidas estándares por semana
	• Estar en riesgo de sufrir consecuencias negativas en la salud y en la vida social
Abuso de Alcohol o Dependencia	• El consumo excesivo ha producido una necesidad física de alcohol o ha conllevado a otros problemas

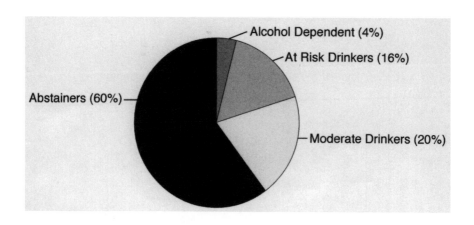

5ª PARTE: CONSECUENCIAS DEL CONSUMO RIESGOSO Y DE LOS PROBLEMAS CON EL ALCOHOL

Consumir alcohol puede afectar su *salud física, bienestar social, y emocional así como sus relaciones personales.*

Los siguientes son algunos de los efectos positivos que a veces se atribuyen al consumo de alcohol. Marquemos aquellos que usted cree que aplican en su caso.

☐ Euforia temporaria
☐ Relajación
☐ Evitar sensaciones de incomodidad

☐ Olvidar problemas
☐ Sensación de autoconfianza
☐ Se le hace más fácil el exponer sus puntos de vista a otros

☐ Se disfruta el sabor
☐ Disminución temporal de estrés

☐ Facilita las relaciones sociales

Las siguientes son algunas de las *consecuencias negativas* que se pueden atribuir al consumo de alcohol. Marquemos aquellos problemas que le afecten a usted, independientemente de que usted crea que estén relacionados con el consumo de alcohol.

☐ Dificultad para manejar situaciones estresantes
☐ Problemas para dormir
☐ Accidentes/caídas

☐ Depresión
☐ Problemas de memoria o confusión
☐ Problemas para relacionarse con otros

☐ Pérdida de independencia
☐ Desnutrición
☐ Aumento en el riesgo de ser agredido/a o atacado/a

☐ Problemas en actividades comunitarias
☐ Reducción de la eficacia de las medicinas
☐ Problemas económicos

☐ Alta presión sanguínea
☐ Aumento en los efectos secundarios de las medicinas
☐ Dolor de estómago

☐ Problemas de funcionamiento sexual
☐ Problemas con el hígado

6ª PARTE: RAZONES PARA DISMINUIR O ELIMINAR EL CONSUMO DE ALCOHOL

El propósito de este paso es pensar en la mejor razón que exista para disminuir o eliminar su consumo de alcohol. Las razones serán distintas para diferentes personas.

La siguiente lista identifica algunas de las razones por las que algunas personas deciden disminuir o eliminar el consumo de alcohol. Ponga una X en el recuadro que corresponde a las tres razones que usted considera más importantes por las que quisiera disminuir o eliminar el consumo de alcohol. A lo mejor se le ocurren otras razones que no estén en la lista.

□ Consumir menos calorías sin valor nutritivo (las bebidas alcohólicas contienen muchas calorías.
□ Dormir major
□ Mantener la independencia
□ Sentirse mejor
□ Ahorrar dinero
□ Ser más feliz
□ Reducir la posibilidad de resultar herido/a en un accidente de tránsito
□ Tener mejores relaciones familiares
□ Participar más en actividades comunitarias
□ Tener mejores amistades
□ Otras: _____

Escriba aquí las tres razones más importantes por las cuales usted elige reducir o eliminar el consumo de alcohol:

1._____

2._____

3._____

Piense en las consecuencias de seguir consumiendo alcohol en exceso. Ahora piense en cómo su vida podría mejorar si decidiera cambiar sus hábitos al reducir o eliminar el consumo de alcohol. Cuáles serían los beneficios obtenidos en cuanto a…?

La salud física:

La salud mental:

La familia:

Las otras relaciones:

Las actividades:

7ª PARTE: CONTRATO DE CONSUMO DE BEBIDAS ALCOHOLICAS

El propósito de este paso es poner un límite a su consumo de bebidas alcohólicas por un periodo de tiempo específico. Hable con su doctor para llegar a acuerdo en cuanto a una meta razonable. Para algunas personas una meta razonable sería abstenerse o no consumir bebidas alcohólicas.

A medida que desarrolle este contrato, conteste las siguientes preguntas:

- ¿Cuántas bebidas estándares?
- ¿Cada cuánto?
- ¿Por cuánto tiempo?

CONTRATO DE CONSUMO DE BEBIDAS ALCOHOLICAS

Fecha _____

Firma del paciente _____

Firma del clínico _____

TARJETA DE BEBIDAS DIARIAS

Llevar la cuenta de cuánto toma se puede hacer usando las tarjetas de bebidas diarias. Se utiliza una tarjeta por semana. Escriba el número de bebidas que toma todos los días. Al final de la semana sume el número total de bebidas que ha tomado durante la semana.

TARJETA DIARIA

LLEVE UN REGISTRO DE LO QUE TOMA EN LOS PROXIMOS 7 DIAS

FECHA DE COMIENZO _____

	Cerveza	Vino	Licor	Número
Domingo				
Lunes				
Martes				
Miércoles				
Jueves				
Viernes				
Sábado				
			Total semanal:	

LLEVE UN REGISTRO DE LO QUE TOMA EN LOS PROXIMOS 7 DIAS

FECHA DE COMIENZO _____

	Cerveza	Vino	Licor	Número
Domingo				
Lunes				
Martes				
Miércoles				
Jueves				
Viernes				
Sábado				
			Total semanal:	

8ª PARTE: MANEJAR SITUACIONES DE RIESGO

El deseo de beber puede cambiar de acuerdo a su estado de ánimo, las personas con las que está, y la disponibilidad del alcohol. Piensa en la última veces que tomó una alcohol.

A continuación tiene ejemplos de situaciones de riesgo. La siguiente lista le puede ayudar a recordar situaciones que puedan resultar en el consumo riesgoso.

- Reuniones familiares
- Aburrimiento
- Tensión

- No poder dormir
- Familia
- Amigos

- Rabia
- Ver televisión
- Ver tomar a los demás

- Sentirse solo/a
- Sentimientos de fracaso
- Frustración
- Uso de tabaco

- Críticas
- Fiestas/cenas

- Hijos y nietos
- Anucios de TV o de revistas

- Ciertos lugares
- Después de las actividades diarias
- Fines de semana
- Discusiones

¿Cuáles son las situaciones que le hacen querer tomar a un nivel riesgoso? Por favor escríbalas aquí:

1. _____

2. _____

Maneras de Lidiar Con Situaciones de Riesgo

Es importante hallar una manera de asegurarse de no vaya a pasarse de los límites de consumo cuando sienta la tentación. Aquí tiene algunos ejemplos:

- Llamar a un amigo por teléfono
- Salir a caminar

- Llamar a un vecino
- Ver una película

- Leer un libro
- Participar en una actividad que disfrute

Es posible que algunas de estas ideas no funcionen para usted, pero otros métodos de lidiar con situaciones de riesgo podrían servirle. Identifique algunas técnicas que usted podría usar para manejar las situaciones de riesgo específicas que usted mencionó anteriormente.

1. Para la primera situación o sentimiento de riesgo, escriba algunas técnicas que podría usar para lidiar con ella.

_____

_____

2. Para la segunda situación o sentimiento de riesgo, escriba algunas técnicas que podría usar para lidiar con ella.

_____

_____

Piense en otras situaciones y maneras de lidiar con ellas sin hacer uso del alcohol.

9ª PARTE: RESUMEN DE LA VISITA

Hoy hemos abarcado mucha información. Cambiar el comportamiento, especialmente los patrones de consumir alcohol, puede ser un reto difícil. Los siguientes puntos pueden ayudarle a seguir con este nuevo comportamiento y a mantener el acuerdo para limitar el consumo, especialmente durante las primeras semanas cuando es más difícil. Recuerde que usted está cambiando un hábito, y esto puede ser una tarea difícil. Con el tiempo se vuelve más fácil.

- Recuerde su meta de limitar el consumo:_____
- Lea este cuaderno frecuentemente.
- Cada vez que siente la tentación de exceder los límites y logra resistirse, felicítese por que está rompiendo con un viejo hábito.
- Si en algún momento se siente muy incómodo/a, recuerde que la sensación va a pasar.
- Al final de cada semana, piense en cuántos días ha podido abstenerse (no consumir alcohol) o ha tomado poco o moderadamente.
- Hay días en que uno consume demasiado alcohol. Si le sucede a usted, NO SE DE POR VENCIDO/A. Simplemente, comience de nuevo al día siguiente.
- No dude en llamar a su médico si necesita ayuda o en caso de emergencia.

GRACIAS POR PROBAR ESTE PROGRAMA.

Por favor traiga sus tarjetas de bebidas diarias a su próxima visita para revisarlas con la enfermera y/o con su médico.

Appendix J

Health Promotion Workbook for Older Adults: Follow-up Session–Spanish Version

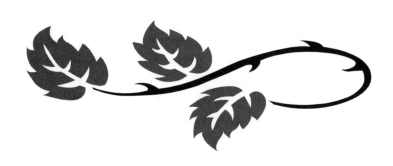

Health Promotion Workbook
For Older Adults:
Follow-up Session–Spanish
Version

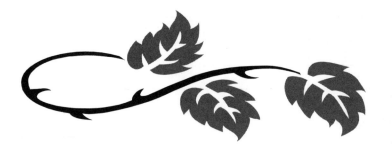

Fecha de hoy ___/___/___

1ª PARTE: PROPOSITO DE LA VISITA DE HOY

En su visita inicial hablamos acerca de cómo el consumo de alcohol puede afectar la salud y el bienestar en general. Al concluir la visita, usted firmó un contrato sobre el consumo de alcohol y aceptó que nos reuniéramos otra vez para hablar de su consumo de alcohol desde entonces.

Hoy, vamos a ver cuánto ha estado tomando desde nuestra última visita y modificar o reveer su meta con respecto al consumo de alcohol.

2ª PARTE: REPASO DE SU CONSUMO DE ALCOHOL

Vamos a comenzar revisando las tarjetas de bebidas alcohólicas diarias de su última visita.

Si no las tiene o no pudo completarlas, sigamos adelante.

Veamos cuánto ha tomado usted durante la última semana.

QUE HA TOMADO EN LOS ULTIMOS SIETE DIAS?

FECHA DE COMIENZO _____

	Cerveza	Vino	Licor	Número
Domingo				
Lunes				
Martes				
Miércoles				
Jueves				
Viernes				
Sábado				
			Total semanal:	

3ª PARTE: REPASO DE LOS CAMBIOS EN EL CONSUMO DE ALCOHOL

De acuerdo a su diario de consumo,   □ ha disminuido?
¿su uso de alcohol...   □ ha permanecido igual?
                                          □ ha aumentado?
¿Cumplió usted con la meta que se había fijado en nuestra última
reunión?   □ No
                                     □ Sí

Ahora hablemos de aquellos días en los cuales usted trató de
reducir o eliminar el consumo de alcohol, aunque no haya
logrado hacerlo. Cuénteme las veces en que usted trató o logró
de reducir o eliminar el consumo. Anote las ocasiones en que
usted intentó o dejó de beber.

1. _____

_____

2. _____

_____

3. _____

_____

¿Encontró usted difícil tratar de disminuir el consumo de alcohol?
                                     □ No
                                     □ Sí
De ser así, ¿qué se le hizo difícil?

1. _____

2. _____

3. _____

Si logró disminuir el consumo, ¿Hubo algún aspecto positivo
al lograrlo?   □ No
De ser así, ¿cuáles fueron las cosas positivas?   □ Sí

1. _____

2. _____

3. _____

4ª PARTE: CONSECUENCIAS DEL CONSUMO RIESGOSO Y DE LOS PROBLEMAS CON EL ALCOHOL

Como hablamos la última vez, consumir alcohol puede afectar *su salud física, bienestar emocional y social, así como sus relaciones personales.*

Vamos a mencionar algunos de los efectos positivos que, a veces, se atribuyen al consumo de alcohol. Marquemos aquéllos que usted cree que aplican en su caso.

☐ Euforia temporaria   ☐ Relajación   ☐ Evitar sensaciones de incomodidad

☐ Olvidar los problemas   ☐ Sensación de autoconfianza   ☐ Se le hace más fácil el exponer su puntos de vista a otros

☐ Se disfruta el sabor
☐ Le facilita sus relaciones sociales   ☐ Disminución temporal de estrés

Si usted modificó el consumo, ¿ha notado cambios buenos o malos en alguna de estas áreas? Si usted disminuyó el consumo, ¿ha notado alguno de estos efectos?

A continuación tenemos algunas de las *consecuencias negativas* del consumo de alcohol. Marquemos aquellos problemas que le afectan a usted, idependientemente de que usted crea que están relacionados con el consumo de alcohol.

☐ Dificultad para manejar situaciones estresantes   ☐ Problemas para dormir   ☐ Accidentes/caídas

☐ Depresión   ☐ Problemas de memoria o confusión   ☐ Problemas para relacionarse con otros

☐ Pérdida de independencia   ☐ Desnutrición   ☐ Aumento en el riesgo de ser agredido/a o atacado/a

☐ Problemas en actividades comunitarias   ☐ Reducción de la eficacia de las medicinas   ☐ Problemas económicos

☐ Alta presión sanguínea   ☐ Aumento en los efectos secundarios de las medicinas   ☐ Dolor de estómago

☐ Problemas de funcionamiento sexual   ☐ Problemas con el hígado

¿Alguna de estas áreas ha mejorado o ha empeorado desde su última visita? Modificar el consumo, ¿afectó alguna de estas áreas?

5ª PARTE: RAZONES PARA DISMINUIR O ELIMINAR EL CONSUMO DE ALCOHOL

Revisaremos las razones que usted identificó para disminuir o eliminar el consumo de alcohol. Primero, vamos a marcar las razones para disminuir o eliminar el consumo que USTED eligió la primera vez que nos reunimos. ¿Ha cambiado alguna de ellas? ¿Cuál de ellas le gustaría marcar esta vez?

	Selecciones anteriores	Razones actuales
Consumir menos calorías sin valor nutritivo (las bebidas alcohólicas contienen muchas calorías)	☐	☐
Dormir mejor	☐	☐
Mantener la independencia	☐	☐
Sentirse mejor	☐	☐
Ahorrar dinero	☐	☐
Ser más feliz	☐	☐
Reducir la posibilidad de resultar herido /a en un accidente de tránsito	☐	☐
Tener mejores relaciones familiares	☐	☐
Participar más en actividades comunitarias	☐	☐
Tener mejores amistades	☐	☐
Mejorar su salud	☐	☐
Otras:_____	☐	☐

6ª PARTE: CONTRATO DE CONSUMO DE ALCOHOL

Queremos rever su decisión de reducir el consumo de alcohol y de fijar un límite de consumo. Hable con su doctor para llegar a un acuerdo en cuanto a una meta razonable. Para algunas personas una meta razonable sería abstenerse o no consumir bebidas alcohólicas.

A medida que desarrolle este contrato, conteste las siguientes preguntas:

- ¿Cuántas bebidas estándares?
- ¿Cada cuánto?
- ¿Durante cuánto tiempo?

CONTRATO DE CONSUMO DE BEBIDAS ALCOHOLICAS

Fecha_____

Firma del paciente _____

Firma del clínico _____

Las bebidas que aparecen a continuación, en tamaño normal, contienen básicamente la misma cantidad de alcohol puro. Se puede pensar en cada una como una bebida estándar.

¿Que constituye una bebida estándar?
un bebida estándar equivale =

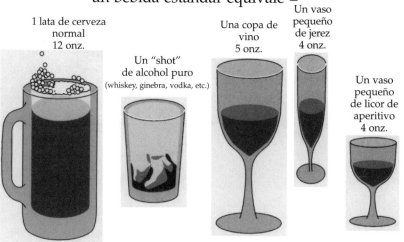

1 lata de cerveza normal 12 onz.

Un "shot" de alcohol puro (whiskey, ginebra, vodka, etc.)

Una copa de vino 5 onz.

Un vaso pequeño de jerez 4 onz.

Un vaso pequeño de licor de aperitivo 4 onz.

7ª PARTE: MANERAS DE LIDIAR CON SITUACIONES DE RIESGO

Es importante hallar una manera de asegurarse de no vaya a pasarse de los límites de consumo cuando sienta la tentación. Aquí tiene algunos ejemplos:

- Llamar a un amigo por teléfono
- Salir a caminar
- Llamar a un vecino
- Ver una película
- Leer un libro
- Participar en una actividad que disfrute

Es posible que algunas de estas ideas no funcionen para usted, pero otros métodos de lidiar con situaciones de riesgo podrían servirle. Identifique algunas técnicas que usted podría usar para manejar situaciones de riesgo específicas.

¿Cuáles técnicas ha probado? ¿Le funcionaron o no? ¿Por qué?

1. _____

_____

2. _____

_____

3. _____

_____

¿Cuáles son algunas de las cosas que le gustaría tratar o continuar haciendo para ayudar a reducir su consumo de alcohol o para mantener la meta que ha alcanzado?

1. _____

_____

2. _____

_____

3. _____

_____

Piense en otras situaciones y técnicas que podría usar para lidiar con ellas sin hacer uso del alcohol.

8ª PARTE: RESUMEN DE LA VISITA

Hoy hemos abarcado mucha información. Cambiar el comportamiento, especialmente los patrones de consumo de alcohol, puede ser un reto difícil. Los siguientes puntos pueden ayudarle a seguir con este nuevo comportamiento y a mantener el acuerdo para limitar el consumo, especialmente durante las primeras semanas cuando es más difícil. Recuerde que usted está cambiando un hábito, y esto puede ser una tarea difícil. Con el tiempo se vuelve más fácil.

- Recuerde su meta de limitar el consumo:_____
- Lea este cuaderno frecuentemente.
- Cada vez que siente la tentación de exceder los límites y logra resistirse, felicítese por que está rompiendo con un viejo hábito.
- Si en algún momento se siente muy incómodo/a, recuerde que la sensación va a pasar.
- Al final de cada semana, piense en cuantos días ha podido abstenerse (no consumir alcohol) o ha tomado poco o moderadamente.
- Hay días en que uno consume demasiado alcohol. Si le sucede a usted, NO SE DE POR VENCIDO/A. Simplemente, comience de nuevo al día siguiente.
- No dude en llamar a su médico si necesita ayuda o en caso de emergencia.

GRACIAS POR PROBAR ESTE PROGRAMA.

Por favor traiga sus tarjetas de bebidas diarias a su próxima visita para revisarlas con la enfermera y/o con su médico.

TARJETA DE BEBIDAS DIARIAS

Nos gustaría que usted continuara llevando un registro de su consumo de alcohol usando las tarjetas de bebidas diarias. Se usa una tarjeta por semana. Cada día escriba el número de bebidas que ha tomado. Al final de la semana sume el número total de bebidas que ha tomado durante la semana.

TARJETA DIARIA

LLEVA EL RECORD DE LO QUE TOMA EN LOS PROXIMOS 7 DIAS

FECHA DE COMIENZO _____

	Cerveza	Vino	Licor	Número
Domingo				
Lunes				
Martes				
Miércoles				
Jueves				
Viernes				
Sábado				
			Total semanal:	

LLEVA EL RECORD DE LO QUE TOMA EN LOS PROXIMOS 7 DIAS

FECHA DE COMIENZO _____

	Cerveza	Vino	Licor	Número
Domingo				
Lunes				
Martes				
Miércoles				
Jueves				
Viernes				
Sábado				
			Total semanal:	

LLEVA EL RECORD DE LO QUE TOMA EN LOS PROXIMOS 7 DIAS

FECHA DE COMIENZO _____

	Cerveza	Vino	Licor	Número
Domingo				
Lunes				
Martes				
Miércoles				
Jueves				
Viernes				
Sábado				
			Total semanal:	

LLEVA EL RECORD DE LO QUE TOMA EN LOS PROXIMOS 7 DIAS
FECHA DE COMIENZO _____

	Cerveza	Vino	Licor	Número
Domingo				
Lunes				
Martes				
Miércoles				
Jueves				
Viernes				
Sábado				
			Total semanal:	

References

Adams, W. L. (1995). Interactions between alcohol and other drugs. *International Journal of the Addictions, 30*(13–14), 1903–1923.

Babor, T., & Grant, M. (1992). *Project on identification and management of alcohol-related problems. Report on Phase II: A randomized clinical trial of brief interventions in primary health care.* Geneva: World Health Organization.

Blow, F. (1998). *Substance abuse among older americans* (DHHS No. (SMA) 98–3179). Washington, DC: U.S. Government Printing Office.

Blow, F., & Barry, K. (in press). Brief interventions. *Journal of Geriatric Psychiatry and Neurology.*

Broe, G. A., Creasey, H., Jorm, A. F., Bennett, H. P., Casey, B., Waite, L. M., & Grayson. (1998). Health habits and risk of cognitive impairment and dementia. *Australian and New Zealand Journal of Public Health, 22*(5), 621–623.

Buchsbaum, D. G., Buchanan, R., Welsh, J., Centor, R., & Schnoll, S. (1992). Screening for drinking disorders in the elderly using the CAGE questionnaire. *Journal of the American Geriatric Society, 40*, 662—665.

Council on Scientific Affairs. (1996). Alcohol and the driver. *Journal of the American Medical Association, 255*, 522—527.

Dufour, M. C., Archer, L., & Gordis, E. (1992). Alcohol and the elderly. *Clinics in Geriatric Medicine, 8*, 127—141.

Ensrud, K. E., Nevitt, M. C., Yunis, C., Cauley, J. A., Seeley, D. G., Fox, K. M., & Cummings, S. R. (1994). Correlates of Impaired Function in Older Women. *Journal of the American Geriatrics Society, 42*, 481—489.

Ewing, J. A. (1984). Detecting alcoholism: The CAGE questionnaire. *Journal of the American Medical Association, 252*, 1905—1907.

Fleming, M., Manwell, L., Barry, K., & Adams, W. (1999). Brief physician advice for alcohol problems in older adults: a randomized community-based trial. *Journal of Family Practice, 48*, 378—84.

Fleming M, C. (1999). *A Guide to Substance Abuse Services for Primary Care Clinicians.* Washington, DC: U.S. Government Printing Office.

Fleming, M. F., Barry, K. L., Manwell, L. B., Johnson, K., & London, R. (1997). Brief physician advice for problem alcohol drinkers. *Journal of the American Medical Association, 277*, 1039—1045.

Fraser, A. G. (1997). Pharmacokinetic interactions between alcohol and other drugs. *Clinical Pharmacokinetics, 33*(2), 79–90.

Gales, B. J., & Menard, S. M. (1995). Relationship between the administration of selected medications and falls in hospitalized elderly patients. *Annals of Pharmacotherapy, 29*(4), 354–358.

Goldberg, D. (1978). *Manual of the General Health Questionnaire.* Windsor, England: National Foundation for Educational Research.

Graham, K., & Schmidt, G. (1999). Alcohol use and psychosocial well-being among older adults. *Journal of Studies on Alcohol, 60,* 345—351.

Habraken, H., Soenen, K., Blondeel, L., Van Elsen, J., Bourda, J., Coppens, E., & Willeput, M. (1997). Gradual withdrawal from benzodiazepines in residents of homes for the elderly: experience and suggestions for future research. *European Journal of Clinical Pharmacology, 51*(5), 355–358.

Hamilton, M. (1960). A rating scale for depression. *Journal of Neurology, Neurosurgery, and Psychiatry, 23,* 56—65.

Hansagi, H., Romelsjo, A., Gerhardsson, M., Andreasson, S., & Leifman, A. (1995). Alcohol consumption and stroke mortality 20-year followup of 15,077 men and women. *Stroke, 26,* 1768—1773.

Hasegawa, K., Mukasa, H., Nakazawa, Y., Kodama, H., & Nakamura, K. (1990). Primary and secondary depression in alcoholism–clinical features and family history. *Drug and Alcohol Dependence, 27,* 275—281.

Hemmelgarn, B., Suissa, S., Huang, A., Boivin, J. F., & Pinard, G. (1997). Benzodiazepine use and the risk of motor vehicle crash in the elderly [see comments]. *Journal of the American Medical Association, 278*(1), 27–31.

Herings, R. M. C., Stricker, B. H. C., deBoer, A., Bakker, A., & Sturmans, F. (1995). Benzodiazepines and the risk of falling leading to femur fractures. *Archives of Internal Medicine, 155,* 1801—1807.

Holroyd, S., & Duryee, J. (1997). Substance use disorders in a geriatric psychiatry outpatient clinic: prevalence and epidemiologic characteristics. *Journal of Nervous and Mental Disease, 185*(10), 627–632.

Hylek, E. M., Heiman, H., Skates, S. J., Sheehan, M. A., & Singer, D. E. (1998). Acetaminophen and other risk factors for excessive warfarin anticoagulation. *Journal of the American Medical Association, 279*(9), 657–662.

Jones, T. V., lndsey, B. A., Yount, P., Soltys, R., & Farani-enayat, B. (1993). Alcoholism screening questions: Are they valid in elderly medical outpatients. *Journal of General Internal Medicine, 8,* 674—678.

Kadden, R., Carroll, K., Donovan, D., Cooney, N., Monti, P., Abrams, D., Litt, M., & Hester, R. (Eds.). (1995). *Cognitive Behavioral Coping Skills Therapy Manual: A Clinical Research Guide for Therapists Treating Individuals with Alcohol Abuse and Dependence.* Rockville, MD: National Institutes of Health.

Kivela, S. L., Nissinen, A., & Ketola, A. (1989). Alcohol consumption and mortality in aging or aged Finnish men. *Journal of Clinical Epidemiology, 42,* 61—68.

Klatsky, A. L., Armstrong, M. A., & Friedman, G. D. (1990). Risk of cardiovascular mortality in alcohol drinkers, ex-drinkers and nondrinkers. *American Journal of Cardiology, 66,* 1237—1242.

LaCroix, A. Z., Guralnik, J. M., Berkman, L. F., Wallace, R. B., & Satterfield, S. (1993). Maintaining mobility in late life. *Journal of Epidemiology, 137,* 858—869.

Miller, W., & Rollnick, S. (1991). *Motivational Interviewing: Preparing People to Change Addictive Behavior.* New York: Guilford Press.

Morton, J. L., Jones, T. V., & Manganaro, M. A. (1996). Performance of alcoholism screening questionnaires in elderly veterans. *American Journal of Medicine, 101,* 153—159.

Nelson, D. E., Sattin, R. W., Langlois, J. A., DeVito, C. A., & Stevens, J. A. (1992). Alcohol as a risk factor for fall injury events among elderly persons living in the community. *Journal of the American Geriatrics Society, 40,* 658—661.

Nelson, H. D., Nevitt, M. C., Scott, J. C., Stone, K. L., & Cummings, S. R. (1994). Smoking, alcohol, and neuromuscular and physical function of older women. *Journal of the American Medical Association, 272*(23), 1825—1831.

Newman, A., Enright, P., Manolio, T., Haponik, E., & Whal, P. (1997). Sleep disturbances, psyhcosocial correlates, and cardiovascular disease in 5,201 older adults: The cardiovasular health study. *Journal of the American Geriatrics Society, 45,* 1—7.

O'Loughlin, J. L., Robitaille, Y., Boivin, J.-F., & Suissa, S. (1993). Incidence of and risk factors for falls and injurious falls among the community-dwelling elderly. *American Journal of Epidemiology, 137,* 342—354.

Orgogozo, J. M., Dartigues, J. F., Lafont, S., Letenneur, L., Commenges, D., & Salamon. (1997). Wine consumption and dementia in the elderly: a prospective. *Revue Neurologique, 153*(3), 185–192.

Oslin, D., Katz, I., Edell, W., & TenHave, T. (in press). The effects of alcohol consumption on the treatment of depression among the elderly. *American Journal of Geriatric Psychiatry.*

Oslin, D., Liberto, J., O'Brien, J., Krois, S., & Norbeck, J. (1997). Naltrexone as an adjunctive treatment for older patients with alcohol dependence. *American Journal of Geriatric Psychiatry, 5,* 324—332.

Oslin, D.W., Pettinati, H.M., Luck, G., Semwanga, A., Cnaan, A., & O'Brien, C.P. (1998). Clinical correlations with carbohydrate-deficient transferrin levels in women with alcoholism. *Alcoholism, Clinical and Experimental Research, 22*(9), 1981–1985.

Radloff, L. (1977). The CES-D scale: A self-report depression scale for research in the general population. *Applied Psychological Measurement, 1,* 385—401.

Rickels, K., Case, W. G., Schweizer, E., Garcia-Espana, F., & Fridman, R. (1991). Long-term benzodiazepine users 3 years after participation in a discontinuation program. *American Journal of Psychiatry, 148*(6), 757–761.

Ried, L. D., Lohnson, R. E., & Gettman, D. A. (1998). Benzodiazepine exposure and functional status in older people. *Journal of the American Geriatric Society, 46,* 71—76.

Rimm, E. B., Giovannucci, E. L., Willett, W. C., Colditz, G. A., Ascherio, A., Rosner, B., & Stampfer, M. J. (1991). Prospective study of alcohol consumption and risk of coronary disease in men. *Lancet, 338,* 464—468.

Salaspuro, M. (1994). Biological state markers of alcohol abuse. *Alcohol Health and Research World, 18*(2), 131–135.

Saunders, J. B., Asland, O. G., Babor, T. F., Delafuente, J. R., & Grant, M. (1993). Development of the alcohol-use disorders identification test (AUDIT)–WHO collaborative project on early detection of persons with harmful alcohol-consumption. *Addiction, 88,* 791—804.

Saunders, P. A., Copeland, J. R., Dewey, M. E., Davidson, I. A., McWilliam, C., Sharma, V., & Sullivan, C. (1991). Heavy drinking as a risk factor for depression and dementia in elderly men. *British Journal of Psychiatry, 159,* 213—216.

Schuckit, M. A., Tipp, J. E., Bergman, M., Reich, W., Hesselbrock, V. M., & Smith, T. L. (1997). Comparison of induced and independent major depressive disorders in 2,945 alcoholics. *American Journal of Psychiatry, 154,* 948—957.

Schwab, J. J., Bialow, M., Clemmons, R., et al. (1967). The Beck Depression Inventory in medical inpatients. *Act Psychiatrica Scandinavia, 43,* 255—266.

Schweizer, E., Case, W. G., & Rickels, K. (1989). Benzodiazepine dependence and withdrawal in elderly patients. *American Journal of Psychiatry, 146*(4), 529–531.

Simon, G. E., VonKorff, M., Barlow, W., Pabiniak, C., & Wagner, E. (1996). Predictors of chronic benzodiazepine use in a health maintenance organization sample. *Journal of Clinical Epidemiology, 49*(9), 1067–1073.

Stampfer, M. J., Colditz, G. A., Willett, W. C., Speizer, F. E., & Hennekens, C. H. (1988). A prospective study of moderate alcohol consumption and the risk of coronary disease and stroke in women. *New England Journal of Medicine, 319,* 267—273.

Sullivan, J. T., Sykora, K., Schneiderman, J., & Naranjo, C. A. (1989). Assessment of alcohol withdrawal: the revised clinical institute withdrawal. *British Journal of Addiction, 84*(11), 1353–1357.

Tsuang, D., Cowley, D., Ries, R., Dunner, D. L., & Roy-Byrne, P. P. (1995). The effects of substance use disorder on the clinical presentation of anxiety and depression in an outpatient psychiatric clinic. *Journal of Clinical Psychiatry, 56,* 549—555.

Wagman, A. M., Allen, R. P., & Upright, D. (1977). Effects of alcohol consumption upon parameters of ultradian sleep rhythms in alcoholics. *Advances in Experimental Medicine and Biology, 85A,* 601—616.

Willett, W. C., Stampfer, M. J., Colditz, G. A., Rosner, B. A., Hennekens, C. H., & Speizer, F. E. (1987). Moderate alcohol consumption and the risk of breast cancer. *New England Journal of Medicine, 316,* 1174—1189.

Index

Springer Publishing Company

Emotional Problems in Later Life, 2nd Edition
Intervention Strategies for Professional Caregivers

Dan Blazer, MD, PhD

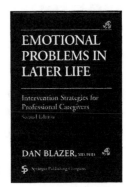

Written by an internationally renowned authority in geriatric psychiatry, this text deals with the most common emotional problems affecting the elderly — memory loss, depression, anxiety, sleeping problems, alcohol and drug abuse, and others.

Highlights:

- The nature and scope of the problem
- The etiological factors involved
- A diagnostic workup
- Treatment strategies

This new edition has been updated to include financing health care for older adults. An invaluable reference for all who work with this challenging, underserved, and rapidly growing aged population.

Partial Contents:

Preface: Who are the Elderly? • Communicating with the Older Adult Suffering Emotional Problems • Memory Loss • Depression • Suspiciousness and Agitation • Anxiety • Hypochondriasis and Other Somatoform Disorders • Sleeping Problems • Alcohol and Drug Abuse • Emotional Problems Associated with Physicial Illness • Bereavement • Working with the Family of the Older Adult Suffering Emotional Problems • Successful Aging • Financing the Care for Emotional Problems in Later Life

1997   280pp   0-8261-7561-9   hardcover $39.95   (outside US $45.80)

536 Broadway, New York, NY 10012-3955 • (212) 431-4370 • Fax (212) 941-7842
Order Toll-Free: (877) 687-7476 • Order on-line: www.springerpub.com

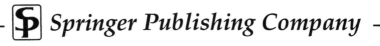